THE HEAL YOURSELF

Home Handbook of

UNUSUAL REMEDIES

Also by the Authors

NATURE'S 12 MAGIC HEALERS:
THE AMAZING SECRETS OF CELL SALTS

THE HEAL YOURSELF
Home Handbook of
UNUSUAL REMEDIES

Lionel Rolfe

and Nigey Lennon

Parker Publishing Company, Inc.
West Nyack, New York

Library of Congress Cataloging in Publication Data

Rolfe, Lionel
  The heal yourself home handbook of unusual remedies.

  Includes index.
  1. Therapeutics—Popular works.   2. Self-care,
Health. I. Lennon, Nigey   . II. Title.
RM122.5.R64   1983   615.8'8   82-14274
ISBN 0-13-384685-7
      0-13-384677-6 {PBK}

Printed in the United States of America

A WORD FROM THE AUTHORS

A few years ago our friend, writer and editor Dorothy Schuler, moved to a hidden house at the end of a canyon in the Hollywood hills. Going to visit her was a tonic, for it was like taking a relaxing trip to the country. On hot summer nights, we'd sit with Dorothy and her husband Robert and look at the stars. Because they lived at the end of a street that had no street lighting, and because the house was nestled at the bottom of a deep canyon whose walls kept out the rest of the city lights, it got very dark and very quiet in their house. The lights of Hollywood only a couple of miles away were gone, as if by magic, as if they belonged to another world, another place and another time. The only sounds were those of the rustling chapparal and crickets and birds, and sometimes cats and dogs, emanating from the darkness. In the surrounding canyon walls was the smell of the chapparal, and on their property itself, came the smells of trees and bushes, ferns and herbs. Dorothy, who had always lived in urban areas, was discovering the joys of growing herbs in her rural oasis there in the urban maelstrom, and had planted them around the property wherever she could find room. Her interest in growing herbs originally began when she was hired to edit a book on herbs, for Dorothy makes her living as a writer and editor. Not only did she grow them, she also began to collect a library on herbal remedies that after several years was

better and more complete than any in the various libraries
around Los Angeles. Eventually, she became involved
with other herbalists, and today she has become quite an
authority (if not in print) among her many friends and
neighbors anxious for her herbal remedies and cosmetics.
Through our association with her, we were drawn into
the fascinating world of herbalism, and we can truly say
that without her this book could not have been written.

Herbs are not the only unusual home remedies we
have compiled for you in this book. In listening to
Dorothy, we discovered many other surprising things
you can do with common items you probably already
have in your kitchen — many of them we unearthed as
our research took us to other times and locations far
beyond Dorothy's library and herb garden. Throughout
our research, we were amazed at how simple some of the
solutions to health complaints can be. Did you know, for
instance, that:

• If you put a fresh raw onion in a glass of hot water,
take it out after a few seconds, add a couple of tablespoons
of California chablis and imbibe it in small quantities
throughout the day, you can banish cold symptoms?

• If you have high blood pressure — as so many of us
in these stressful times do — make sure you consume
dairy products, which include everything from ice
cream to yogurt to just plain milk. The latest scientific
studies indicate that foods such as dairy products, which
contain large amounts of calcium, help reduce high
blood pressure. Says Dr. Jose Villar, professor at the
prestigious Johns Hopkins University, "Our studies
indicate that calcium, the same calcium that you find in
ice cream and other dairy products, does tend to reduce
blood pressure." In a study at the university of 30 men

and women with high blood pressure, a 1,000 milligram tablet of calcium taken daily for 22 weeks reduced the blood pressure by 6 percent in women, and 9 percent in men. By the ounce, ice cream has 24 milligrams of calcium, and whole milk 36.

• If you want to try to stop smoking, here's a remedy that might work. Put a pint of gentian root in a cup of Burgundy wine and water, cover the ingredients in one vessel, and don't touch it for two weeks. If for the next two weeks you take a teaspoon when you first wake up in the morning, one at lunch, one at dinner, and one just before you retire, your desire for tobacco will first lessen, and then just disappear.

• If your eyes are tired, soothe them by placing a slice of cucumber on each lid for five minutes.

• Instead of throwing away that overripe banana, use it as a cosmetic cleanser. It's one of the best there is — it can even lighten age spots and freckles, almost as effectively as grated horseradish.

• Raw potatoes can take away those dark circles under your eyes if you had a rough night; grate and then juice the potatoes and dab on your eyes with cotton balls.

• One of the greatest beauty herbs is aloe vera. If you use an aloe vera gel, you can prevent skin wrinkles and even cure hemorrhoids and peptic ulcers. The milky fluids squeezed from the plant will also heal burns, scrapes and mild abrasions like magic.

• Angelica, a common herb, is just the tonic for heart and lungs.

• Catnip tea, prepared by pouring boiling water on it, and then letting it steep overnight, is a very effective tranquilizer if you can't sleep.

• Chewing ginger root aids digestion. In this book,

you will find myriad such remedies for easily obtainable herbs.

• Raw tomatoes rubbed on the skin work wonders for acne problems.

• Vodka is a great scalp stimulant.

These are just a few of the simple yet unusual methods we have come across to deal with common maladies and problems of our sometimes vulnerable bodies. To discover some of these amazing remedies, many of which you will find on your kitchen shelf or in your supermarket, or in some cases your local health food store, merely turn the page. And again, from the bottom of our hearts, we both thank Dorothy for the world of simple yet unusual remedies which she introduced us to.

Lionel Rolfe and Nigey Lennon

CONTENTS

CONTENTS

CONTENTS

1

HOW EASY-TO-USE,
SIMPLE HOME REMEDIES
WILL KEEP YOU "IN THE PINK"

As nearly everyone is becoming increasingly aware today, the art of staying healthy, and even the art of medicine itself, are just that — art. There are no hard-and-fast rules when it comes to finding cures for dozens of simple, everday ailments such as colds, flu, and headaches. The truth is that modern medicine has yet to improve on the methods known to our ancestors when it comes to dealing with these common yet troublesome ailments; how many times have you heard that, despite all the new developments in "space-age medicine," there is still no cure for the common cold?

Our ancestors certainly didn't have all the answers for these things, either. But whereas we often tend to reach for the most advertised "new and improved" remedy on the drugstore shelf, our forebears employed cures that had been tested, often for many previous centuries, by trial and error. These remedies were not concocted synthetically, and promoted with huge advertising campaigns, but they were taken most often from native plants and similar sources. Other remedies not necessarily from the plant world were also natural — they were simple things like heat and cold, or even that greatest remedy of them all, TLC, Tender Loving Care. The truth is that for a lot of the simple ailments that bother us some-times long-suffering human beings, the old ways were, if not better, at least every bit as good as the new, art-ificial ones on your drugstore shelf.

Becoming knowledgeable about your ailments and how you can safely treat them yourself at home is a good idea, for many reasons. The money you will save in doctors' bills alone is one such good reason, but more importantly, by gaining an understanding of the causes behind simple health problems and how you can treat them, you will be participating fully in the art of stay-ing healthy. An aware, responsible patient tends to be far more successful in dealing with common ailments than a poorly educated one. Then, too, the more you know, the more you will be able to help your doctor if you do need to see him or her, for you will be playing an active rather than a passive role in your health care. This makes things much easier for both you and for your doctor.

FASCINATING REMEDIES

In this book, you will learn about many fascinating remedies for the sort of ailments you can treat yourself. No longer will you need to turn to ineffective, over-the-counter medications when you suffer from colds, flu, headaches, indigestion, insomnia, fatigue and the like. Instead, after reading the book, you should be able to walk into your kitchen and select a safe remedy right off the shelf. Of course as you read this book, you will learn to add items to your shelf you otherwise might not have there — beneficial and health-giving additions. Perhaps you will find the relief you seek in a simple massage. You may even find that your ailment will disappear when you make slight changes in your diet. *Note:* If there is ever any doubt about the nature or severity of a particular health problem, of if symptoms persist even after trying one of the remedies outlined in this book, you should see a doctor as soon as possible.

SIMPLE, BUT EFFECTIVE, REMEDIES: AS OLD AS TIME

King Charlemagne used to hold court in a hot bath because he found it to be a potent remedy for fatigue and insomnia. Science has yet to top that one as a general cure for those two plagues of mankind.

One of medicine's most amazing "wonder drugs," aspirin, is really only a chemically-synthesized version of a willow bark treatment people were using to relieve pain hundreds of years ago.

As you'll see as you read this book, things haven't changed or advanced quite as much as we sometimes like to think they have. You will see how "folk medicine" and "down-home cures" may really be "space-age medicine" in disguise.

SECRETS OF THE FEET

A newspaper in our hometown carried an interview about foot reflexology with Lorayne Krogstad, who runs the Institute of Reflexology in Phoenix, Arizona. The first thing that Krogstad had the reporter do was take off his shoes and socks and clean his feet, first with soap, and then with a squirt or two of Desenex. Then Krogstad took the reporter's right foot in her lap, and began movements like an inchworm with her thumb, tracking from the big toe to the ball of the foot and then sideways.

She asked the reporter if he felt any pain anywhere. "No," he replied. "Does this hurt?" she wanted to know, moving to another part of his foot. To which he responded: "Ouch!"

"I'm finding something — maybe granules in this shoulder," said Krogstad, indicating the reporter's right shoulder. The reporter had to admit that this was pretty insightful, for he had had bursitis there, unmedically attributed to "tennis shoulder" — an ailment of some eighteen years.

TENNIS KNEE CURED

Krogstad also located, between the reporter's third and fourth toes, a bronchial problem. Again the reporter was very impressed, because he had spent a week in bed two months earlier, taking lots of antibiotics in the process of trying to clear up a case of pneumonia. Finally, by feeling around on the outside of his knee, Krogstad found that the reporter had "tennis knee." With some pressure on the area, the reporter found that the pain in the knee diminished considerably; and an hour later, he observed "there was enough pain-free mobility for a sashimi lunch in the lotus position."

The reporter explained in his article that the technique of foot massage, which he called "a 5,000-year-old Oriental refinement of this-little-piggy-went-to-market," is also good for hemorrhoids, arthritis, asthma, sinus problems, insomnia, sciatica and nervous tension, among other things. It is a simple technique that can easily be learned.

TRY SOME PLUG-IN RELIEF
ON YOUR FEET

We laughed when we read the reporter's story, for our experience with foot reflexology has been a little unique. One day half of this duo-writing team complained about how bad her back felt when we were visiting some friends who live in a secluded wooded canyon not far from the sea. Our friends are always full of unusual suggestions, and at the mention of the back problems, they looked at each other with a bit of a sparkle in their eyes, and brought out their electric vibrator. The contraption didn't look very natural — but it also wasn't all that exotic, either. We're not so much against progress we wouldn't try something electric just because it wasn't completely natural. Besides, many drug stores carry them. Anyway, the couple explained that they too suffer from backaches, and a wonderful way to make the whole spinal cord feel better is to run the vibrator along the arch of the foot, from the big toe down to the start of the heel. So the author applied the gizmo to the area on both her feet for as long as she could, and presto, the backache simply vanished.

Our friends explained they had discovered the efficacy of the vibrator applied to the right places on the feet because one suffered from sinus problems, and the other from headaches. In both cases, the point on the bottom of the feet where they applied the vibrator was the same —

the big toe! This was true of both feet. According to our friends, you can get much the same relief by massaging these parts vigorously with your hands — but they insisted that the electric way, in this case, was even better.

STOP SMOKING FOR BACK PAIN

Back pain is universal in the human race, perhaps due to the fact that we homo sapiens are still uncomfortable walking upright — our spines give us nothing but trouble. Despite the numerous operations or medications available in fighting the war against backache, almost nothing works as well as that old-fashioned specific, bed rest — assuming, of course, that you have given foot massage a chance and that wasn't enough. Some eight out of ten people suffer from, and are disabled by, back pain at some point in their lives. It is estimated that the nation spends $5 billion a year for diagnosis and treatment of back pain — yet none of this does as much good as does simple bed rest.

Besides this obvious remedy, however, you can do something else to help your aching back if you are a smoker — you can stop smoking. A University of Vermont study recently revealed that back pains are more frequent among those who smoke, for reasons they weren't entirely sure of. The researchers surmised, however, that apparently "smoker's back" has something to do with the effect of nicotine on the carbon monoxide levels in the blood. This causes the smoker to cough, and the coughing in turn puts an enormous strain on the back itself.

HOW BOB S. FOUND RELIEF
FROM ARTHRITIS

Along the same lines as back pain, although far more painful, is rheumatoid arthritis. Quite accidentally a young camper discovered an effective non-toxic pain reliever. It turned out that this young lad, hardly even a teenager yet, used to suffer terrible arthritis pains when he woke up at night. However, once when Bob S. went camping and spent the night in his sleeping bag, the pain simply was not there. A doctor, intrigued by this discovery, tried the theory of the sleeping bag cure on some hospitalized arthritics. Sure enough, when the patients slept in sleeping bags, they too achieved relief. The reason for the effectiveness of the remedy is that the sleeping bag provides steady and uniform body heat, instead of the alternating hot and cold temperatures that result from sleeping under a carelessly tossed blanket.

A POTPOURRI OF DOWN-HOME
CASES AND REMEDIES

This book will often refer to "down-home" folk remedies, for people in rural areas have traditionally depended on homemade preparations to stave off common ailments in the absence of regular doctors. Some of these remedies are ingenious, and also very effective. If they hadn't worked for people for many generations, we are sure they would not have been passed down from one generation to the next the way they have been.

For Those Painful Hemorrhoids: Many remedies are applied as poultices, which is nothing more than taking the plant medication being used, crushing, grating or chopping it as required, and applying it to the affected area on a clean cloth such as muslin or cotton. The cloth should be slightly dampened, and changed when dry — which usually takes three hours or so. A traditional folk remedy for hemorrhoids is common smoking tobacco and fresh butter applied to the painful area in a poultice. Use one part tobacco to two of butter. The combination should be simmered and strained before application, and it is suggested this remedy be applied two or three times each day. Another hemorrhoid remedy that can bring relief consists of simmering a mixture of one ounce of sulfur, four ounces of hog fat, and half a pint of strong tobacco juice into an ointment, which is then applied to the hemorrhoids. A simpler remedy involves rubbing linseed oil directly onto the external piles.

The gypsy cure for hemorrhoids was more complex. For internal use, an ounce of yellow dock root was boiled in a pint and a half of water. The result was strained, and a wineglass full was taken at night and in the morning. Then an ointment was made from four ounces of pure, unsalted lard, an ounce of plantain leaves, and half an ounce of ground ivy, all common enough herbs to be found in many health food stores. These were placed together in an enamel pan and simmered over low heat for ten minutes, pressing the leaves well into the lard "to get out all the goodness." The resulting mixture was then strained into a jar and left to cool, after which it was applied freely to the rectum at night before retiring. Both the internal and external cures are used simultaneously.

Kidney Problems: Almost all the traditional remedies for kidney problems call for one primary ingredient and it is an ingredient you can find today in nearly every supermarket in the country. That magic ingredient is — hold onto your hats — asparagus. The way you can go about using this remedy is by bruising and splitting the stalk into shreds and then allowing it and the roots to soak in cold water. Strain the resulting liquid and drink the brew at intervals throughout the day. The more you drink of it, the better off you will be.

Shrinking Boils: The peeled off skin of a boiled egg reportedly helps soothe this skin breakout. Just wet the egg skin and apply to the boils. Let remain for a few hours. Better yet, secure with a clean strip of cloth as a bandage and let remain overnight.

Insect in Ear: Try turning the affected ear toward the sun, or a source of bright light if you happen to be indoors. Insects are attracted by light, and will crawl out by themselves. A ripe apple or peach held up near the ear can also tantalize the insect into coming out of your ear, which will be better for you and better for the insect in question for that matter. If all else fails, try pouring a teaspoon of slightly warmed olive oil into your ear. The creature should float right out. If not, fill the ear with warm water plus more olive oil, and that should do the trick.

MARY JANE J.'S INSECT BITE CURE

An Indiana woman, Mary Jane J., remembered as a child having an infected insect bite that was threatening to spread. Her mother washed some leaves from the family's peach tree, mashed them, and applied them to the infected area; then she covered the place with a thin cloth and left it overnight. The next morning the redness and itch were gone, and the area had already begun to heal.

Then there was the New York woman who remembered the advice an old German doctor had given her father when he was suffering from an infection on his face that itched terribly. The doctor suggested to the man that he wash his face with buttermilk and then blot most of it off. The woman said that this remedy worked so well for her father that she herself used buttermilk against acne as a teenager. As a result, she said, even though she was in her seventies at the time, she had not developed any wrinkles.

An old folk remedy for toothache which is still being used by many people today is oil of cloves. You can make it up youself, using the cloves you have in your kitchen, or you can buy it already prepared in increasing numbers of health food stores.

HOW A "WILD TIME" CAN
CURE MELANCHOLY

Spices played a big role in old-time folk remedies and medicines, perhaps because they were convenient and readily available, but also because they worked for many people. Thyme, which was originally called "wilde time" because it was believed to be an aphrodisiac, was also believed by Langham, the early English herbalist, to arrest melancholy. Modern herbalists also believe it has retained similar qualities — a tea made of thyme, for instance, will prevent you from having nightmares.

If you live near a neighborhood where there are Greek stores, you can often find honey made from bees who have dined on thyme, and it is said that the taste and smell are there to enjoy in the honey. To make a tea, make an infusion of an ounce of dry leaves in a pint of boiled water. if there are no Greeks in your area, simply add some other honey to the tea. The result will be almost as good.

YOGURT BATTLES YEAST INFECTIONS

While women may find it a little embarrassing to talk about, the fact is that many seem to suffer from recurrent itching and discharges in and from their vaginas. Another reason that women don't like to talk about these problems is that, despite repeated visits to doctors and one new expensive prescription after another, the problems are just not cleared up. In San Francisco, however, women have banded together and formed various clinics in which they can deal particularly with women-related problems. *(Note:* If the problem persists even after these remedies have been tried, consult a doctor, since the symptoms of other, more serious, ailments can resemble those of a simple vaginal infection.) But some of the women's groups have come up with some ingenious solutions that can be tried in the privacy of your own home.

Douches made from yogurt quite likely were devised a long time ago when some woman with recurrent vaginal itching and discharge made the connection between the lactic acid bacteria, lactobacillus, in yogurt, and her own infection. Yogurt — plain, unflavored yogurt — creates an acid environment in the vagina which makes it less likely to house yeast and annoying bacteria. To use yogurt in this manner, take two tablespoons of plain yogurt and put them in a quart of warm water. Douche with the mixture twice daily, and you can expect the itching and discharge to begin clearing up within two weeks. It is important, however, to use a douche bag, not a syringe douche or expanding bulb-type douche; the douche tip should be finger-shaped and have holes in it. It is also important to keep your douching equipment clean, and never to loan it out to anyone. That is one sure way of spreading infection.

HEALERS FOR ANOTHER IRRITATING "FEMALE" PROBLEM

Trichomonas is a microscopic, one-celled organism usually passed from one partner to another during sexual intercourse. "Trich" flourishes in the vagina, where it causes excessive inflammation and even minor bleeding in severe cases. There is a standard medication used by doctors in the treatment of trichomonas called Flagyl, but it has side effects and can be risky in some cases. However, there are some very effective alternative treatments, and again they have been researched by women's groups in the San Francisco bay area.

One remedy is a chapparal douche — chapparal leaves are common throughout California and parts of the Southwest. You may also be able to purchase them from an herbalist or even a health food store. Take a handful of the chapparal leaves and simmer them in a pint of water for twenty minutes. Let the mixture cool, strain it, and use it as a douche, keeping in mind the instructions above for the proper use of douching equipment. The douche is to be taken twice daily for three consecutive days, or once a day for a week. This treatment can be repeated again, if desired, after waiting a week.

Another useful treatment for "trich" is a garlic suppository. Carefully peel a clove of garlic (but don't leave a nick in the garlic, because it can cause unpleasant burning) and place it in the center of a piece of gauze or cheesecloth. Fold the cloth in half, and twist it around the garlic clove, making a kind of tampon with a gauze tail. Dip the end of the suppository into vegetable oil to facilitate insertion, and insert it into the vagina before going to bed at night. Remove it the next morning on arising. A variation on this same treatment calls for use of the suppository in alternation with a douche made from two tablespoons of white vinegar in a quart of warm water. The treatment should be continued for five days, alternating douche and suppository every other day, with the garlic clove treatment being the first and last remedy used.

Finally, in the case of home treatment for trichomonas, the patient should refrain from sexual intercourse, and she should also increase her water intake to between six and eight glasses a day. A gram of Vitamin C daily is also beneficial in treating such an infection.

HOW LESLIE K. FOUND
RELIEF FROM ASTHMA

Leslie K. was a young woman who lived in New Mexico, where many home remedies have been passed from generation to generation for more than two hundred years. She had moved to Santa Fe from the South in the hope of finding some relief from a persistent case of asthma. One day she discovered an old New Mexico remedy for asthma that called for fig leaves, which were dried and then smoked in a pipe. At first Leslie was extremely skeptical, but after trying this remedy, her asthma disappeared altogether. Now whenever she finds herself becoming short of breath, she resorts to the "dried fig leaf cure," and within minutes she is able to breathe again, even though she now lives in Altadena, California, near Los Angeles, which is a terribly smoggy place since it is located against the mountains of the Los Angeles basin.

RHEUMATISM, EUCALYPTUS AND COD-LIVER OIL

Anyone who has ever suffered from rheumatism (arthritis) knows how agonizing the pain can be. The only suggestion that doctors can make, however, is for the sufferer to take aspirin, or if the pain is unbearable, powerful drugs that often have serious side effects. Here are some alternatives that have worked well for people in the past.

Eucalyptus: Rheumatism and other arthritic conditions have been known to respond well to oil of eucalyptus. The essential oil of this mangy-looking, water-hungry tree is becoming increasingly available in health food stores and some drug stores; or, if you live in California, you will find the eucalyptus to be a very common tree. Oil of eucalyptus is available in liniment form for direct application to sore, aching joints; and eucalyptus teas, which are beneficial for many ailments, are often found at health food stores or herbalists. Or you can make your own liniment by combining crushed eucalyptus leaves with pure olive oil; be sure to limit the amount of eucalyptus leaves used to no more than twenty-five percent of the solution.

Cod-Liver Oil Cure For Arthritis: Another effective remedy for arthritis is, oddly enough, plain cod-liver oil, the stuff you used to hate so much as a child. There is some real scientific evidence that this preparation can ease the pain. Dr. Charles Brusch, medical director of the Brusch Medical Center in Massachussetts, recommends that people suffering from arthritis take two tablespoons of cod-liver oil mixed very well into orange juice or milk. This should be taken on an empty stomach an hour before breakfast, or five hours after dinner. Dr. Brusch reported on the very effective pain-relief achieved with this remedy in a series of experiments published in the *Journal of the National Medical Association* in 1959.

HOW TO LIVE PAST ONE HUNDRED

By now you have probably developed an idea of how easy it is to treat your simple ailments at home with unusual but readily obtainable remedies. But here's something more that is definitely worth pondering. How would you like to live to be more than a hundred years old?

Sounds impossible? It isn't — not necessarily. Recent research shows that it is possible to live much longer lives than we do today, limited only by our genetic tendencies. Some of the important keys to a Methuselan existence include no heavy drinking, no smoking, a diet made up of foods as natural and uncontaminated by chemicals as possible, and plenty of healthful exercise.

But there are other factors as well. People who lead long lives tend to be people who find their work rewarding, who have a high degree of self-esteem, and who live in harmony with the patterns of their environment. That is, their lives are well-ordered, and the pace has a natural rhythm. There is also some interesting evidence to suggest that long-lived people are not in awe of medical advice: they consider it when they need to — they'd be foolish not to. But they also understand that one must take medical advice with more than a grain or two of salt — often doctors just don't know, or what one recommends is entirely contradicted by another, or the treatment may be more damaging than doing nothing at all. Long-lived people also tend to deal with their ailments using natural cures — nutritional and physical therapy sorts of solutions rather than drugs, wherever possible.

With this in mind, you should find this book to be a volume you can treasure throughout your long life. As you have learned from this first chapter, nowadays it is often the natural remedy — the old and proven remedy — which seems the most unusual, and you may wonder how such simple remedies can cure ailments when modern medicine still has very few answers. But this is the very reason these unusual remedies are gaining in popularity. Many people, and often the more intelligent and well-informed ones, are becoming increasingly skeptical about taking a doctor's advice without thinking twice about it. Of course there are times when you should take your physician's word. But so many people have suffered from common ailments and have gone from one doctor to another without finding relief, that it is the simple, old-fashioned, folk-type remedies, such as you will find in this book, that are growing in popularity.

As you use this book, we hope you will gain at least a glimpse into the fascinating horizons of home treatment that are available to you, using remedies right off your kitchen shelf, or which are probably available in your own backyard. Each chapter deals with a particular ailment, or a group of related ailments. Leaf through the book to find what you are looking for. Check the index, too, for the ailment you may be trying to cure.

And remember, better health is right in your hands. You can start right now to help yourself to glowing good health — without side effects, doctors' bills, or potentially dangerous drugs.

That should make you feel better already!

SUMMARY

This chapter introduces you to surprising ways of dealing with common ailments. Oftentimes persons try to deal with these ailments by purchasing over-the-counter remedies though these remedies may actually make the problem worse. Others do nothing at all. The common cold, for instance, has totally eluded treatment by modern scientists. The remedies in this book are derived from the thousands of years of experience human beings have gained in treating their problems with what is available to them. Some of the remedies will surprise you in their simplicity. Most can be easily used in the privacy of your own home. Many use substances that you may already have in your own home.

2

UNCOMMON REMEDIES
FOR THE COMMON COLD

The common cold typifies the kind of ailment that is best treated at home. Although literally no one is exempt from the rigors of runny nose, sore throat, watery eyes and general debility brought on by a cold, modern science has not been able to come up with a cure. Perhaps part of the problem is that a cold can be caused by any one of many different types of virus. Then, too, cold *symptoms* can be brought on by such unrelated causes as nervousness, allergy, attacks of sinusitis, or even marijuana smoking. No wonder that the hunt for an effective cold shot has stopped dead in its tracks — one vaccination simply cannot guarantee the death of such an amorphous malady.

The medicines you can buy over the counter in drug stores are, at best, only of limited effect. If they work at all in suppressing the symptoms of a cold, they also make the cold last that much longer, since there is no way to prevent a cold from running its course. In addition to not curing colds, broad-spectrum antibiotics can also be quite dangerous, since they destroy friendly bacteria along with cold viruses. All of this is made worse by the fact that the common cold appears to be peculiarly affected by one's emotional state, which is why one eminent medical authority, speaking before a Senate hearing, suggested that chicken soup, sympathy and bed rest are still the best medicine for colds.

WHY MOTHER KNEW BEST

When you were a child, your mother probably put you to bed promptly the minute you sneezed or sniffed or exhibited any symptom, however vague, of a cold. You may have resented being immobilized by a seemingly minor ailment, but research is showing that mother probably knew best. Many times, people come down with colds when they are discouraged or tired — and then the treatment for the cold happily coincides with the treatment needed to improve one's mental state. Yet the viruses in question are real enough, and the bed rest doctors recommend for colds is often intended to keep people with colds out of contact with those who don't have them yet. So Mother definitely had the right idea in confining you to quarters when you come down with a cold. Her other specifics, such as chicken soup or hot lemonade, didn't hurt much either.

STEVE W.'S PANTRY SHELF COLD REMEDY

One middle-aged man, Steve W., came down with a cold and discovered that the various cold medicines available over the counter in drug stores were expensive. Worse, the all-night cold medicines that contained a high concentration of alcohol made him much groggier than he liked to be. In addition, he had read that often the only real active ingredient in cold remedies is the alcohol; the sedative effect is what does the most good. Recalling that his wife had some cooking sherry on the pantry shelf, he asked her to make him a cup of camomile tea with two or three tablespoons of sherry just before he turned in. The heat dissipated some of the alcohol's effect, and what was left was enough to do the trick. Sure enough, he slept like a baby, and when he woke up the next morning, he didn't feel half as sluggish as he had when he took the recommended dosage of an all-night cold medication. Plus, he saved himself some money. It didn't take a stroke of genius to come up with this idea, but that's what many common sense home remedies are simple and straightforward.

SIT UP AND BE COUNTED

It's a good idea for a cold sufferer to be propped up on pillows while resting in bed. Otherwise, mucus accumulates in the sinuses. Also, you should remember that coughing serves an important function during a cold. The purpose of coughing is to loosen the secretions that have accumulated in the chest. Thus, cough suppressants are unnecessary and can even be dangerous. In severely stuffy conditions, you might try steam from a kettle or vaporizer. This will loosen up the mucus and enable you to breathe more easily.

L. JOHN HARRIS'S "BEST-SMELLING" COLD SPECIFIC

Both of the authors have long been good friends of L. John Harris, who is the foremost garlic expert in the

41

United States. He is the author of *The Book of Garlic*, which has gone through several printings. In chapter nine, Harris's obsession with garlic is described in a little more detail. But since at the moment we are only concerned with colds, we will say that in all the years we have known Harris, we have never known him to suffer from a cold. In fact, there are times when we are both very much under the weather with a cold, and so is everyone else we know, but Harris just keeps trucking along. During one particularly sniffly season, we decided to take the "garlic cure." Lo and behold, neither of us has suffered from a cold in a long time, either. We're sure, therefore, you will be interested in Harris's cures. The female half of this writing team says she is sure that the increased amount of garlic she has consumed since knowing Harris has helped prevent colds. She quickly adds that she developed a proclivity for garlic. She used to enjoy sandwiches made of nothing but garlic and buttered bread, which she ate not for health reasons but because she likes the taste. However, she also believes that the pungent chili and onions she eats on the hamburgers which she enjoys for many breakfasts must also be given credit for keeping her free of colds.

Coughs: For coughs, Harris boils eleven each of garlic and onion heads in a quart of unpasteurized milk until the vegetables are soft. This mixture should then be strained, and honey added to taste. One tablespoon of this odorous elixir per hour throughout the day is the correct dosage, and it should be taken warm. Harris claims that even the most stubborn cough will loosen up when this mixture is imbibed. He further suggests inhaling the steam from the garlic-onion milk.

Lungs: A quart of boiled water is poured over a pound of fresh garlic which has been cut into slices. Then the mixture is left to stand for 12 hours. After that, honey is added to give the liquid the consistency of syrup. Harris also suggests adding a little vinegar and possibly some caraway seeds or boiled sweet fennel seed to lessen the garlicky odor.

Hoarseness: If you suffer from shortness of breath or from hoarseness during your cold, Harris recommends peeling and slicing garlic cloves into a soup plate. Cover each slice with honey, and in an hour or so a syrup will form, which should be taken in one-teaspoon doses throughout the day.

General Remedies: Harris was single when he wrote this book, and if you're married and don't want to become single, you might consider that before you use these particular cold remedies. Nonetheless, Harris says they are very effective in fighting cold symptoms. What he does is cut cloves of garlic and rub them into the soles of his feet before retiring at night. If he wakes up during the night, he repeats this application of garlic for added effect. During waking hours his variation on this same theme is this: He holds a cut clove of garlic on either side of the mouth, between the cheek and the teeth. The clove should be replaced every few hours. Harris suggests making small cuts in the clove with the teeth in order to release small amounts of garlic juice.

Tightness in the Chest: BRONCHITIS: Garlic cloves are chopped up finely and placed in a pan with equal parts of Vaseline. This mixture is then warmed on the stove until the Vaseline has melted. After stirring, it is allowed to cool. It must not be strained. The resulting paste can be massaged into the chest and back.

Sinus Congestion: Harris recommends chopping up two garlic cloves, adding two ounces of water to them, and stirring the mixture to allow the garlic to settle to the bottom, which will take a few minutes. You should then put a few drops of the liquid into each nostril, sniff, and hold your head back. "This will be very hot but invaluable," Harris reports. It should be repeated several times throughout the day to be fully effective, he adds.

Garlic's effectiveness against colds is something that has been known to folklore for many years, but in recent years there have been more and more scientific studies which also back up garlic's reputation as an effective cold remedy. For example, in one study, it was established that garlic definitely cut short the fever and catarrhal symptoms in thirteen cases of grippe; in twenty-eight cases of sore throat, burning and tickling symptoms were gone only a day after garlic nose drops had been administered — thirty times each day. And in seventy-one cases of clogged and runny noses, a garlic solution taken through the nose and mouth cured all the sufferers in under half an hour!

MIRACULOUS COLD REMEDIES
FROM RUSSIA

Garlic is also highly-favored in the Soviet Union, where it is a time-honored folk remedy against colds and flu. Indeed, garlic is to the Russians what chicken soup is to the Jewish mother and grandmother; it is even known as "Russian Penicillin." There is a good scientific reason for this name — the Russians have produced a medical agent, Allicin, from garlic, reputed to fight both viruses and bacteria. Allicin kills certain unfriendly bacteria, leaving the friendly bacteria untouched. During one recent flu epidemic, the Russians imported five hundred tons of garlic from Europe. They use it in a variety of ways, including topical applications and in vaporized form for cold and bronchial disorders.

In the Soviet Union, there is great emphasis placed on preventative medicine. This is because Soviet hospitals are avoided like the plague; they usually have cramped spaces, lousy food, relatively limited medical attention, and worst of all, modern medicine of a very low quality. Thus, the Russian people have learned to deal with illness outside of their hospitals as much as possible. The traditional Russian grandmother — the "Babushka," — has not given up her traditional remedies of many centuries just because Russian politics changed in 1917. Many of Babushka's cures are concerned with the common cold, as well as with such ailments as rheumatism. Many of these homespun folk remedies are extremely effective, as numerous studies by Russia's medical-scientific establishment have demonstrated. Babushka's remedies have been proven by years and years of successful application in a country where cold climate predisposes its inhabitants to colds, flu and high temperatures.

Babushka's first line of defense is the family diet. Special attention is paid to the vitamins found in fresh, natural foods — vitamin-rich cranberries, pomegranates from Central Asia, and black currants, for example, are eagerly sought out in September. Apples, turnips, and cabbage are staples in the diet because they provide the basic nutrition needed to ward off a cold before it strikes.

The cranberries, pomegranates, and black currants are chopped up raw, conserved with sugar, and eaten like candy "just in case." Berries, garlic, and onions are also consumed as preventatives against the common cold.

That is how Babushka prevents a cold. Once it has struck, however, she looks to her kitchen cupboard for remedies. Tea and raspberry jam are traditional, or a brew of linden leaves with honey is used to bring fever down, while mustard plasters are placed on the chest, and mustard powder is put into thick wool socks on the patient's feet. Mineral water or warm honey mixed with butter is given for the scratchy throat. A quarter of a cup of honey heated in a quarter of a cup of vodka is often given, a tablespoon at a time before meals, to fight coughs. Vodka compresses are used to relieve swollen glands.

The piece de resistance, as noted by one American observer, was the way in which Babushka treats an acutely stuffed-up nose. Her remedy is an onion freshly grated over cotton; two drops of the liquid are put into each nostril. This remedy can "clear the head with explosive force."

SOME OLD-TIME COUGH AND COLD REMEDIES

The Russians are not the only people who have found interesting cough and cold remedies. In the northern and western parts of China, there grows a rather unprepossessing-looking shrub known as "Ma Haung." The Chinese have used this plant for its medicinal value in fighting colds, coughs, and respiratory problems for nearly 5,000 years. Ephedrine, a "miracle drug" used for respiratory ailments, is derived from the Ma Huang plant.

Of course most of us have to seek cold remedies closer to home. Luckily, there are plenty of them. In the small towns and villages of Vermont, a traditional remedy for colds and bronchitis was castor oil mixed with turpentine; the mixture was rubbed liberally on the chest. Honey and apple cider, taken internally or applied topically, together or separately, offer folks in New England quick relief for coughs.

In the Pennsylvania Dutch villages, whenever anyone got a cold or the flu, they were put to bed, covered warmly, and given hot catnip tea with lemon. This induced sweating, lowered the fever, and generally routed the cold. In the Indian homes of Arizona, colds and flu are treated with cedar smoke from wood burned in the fireplaces. The Indians of the Southwest believe that cedar has great powers to fight colds. And in the Ozarks, the popular remedy for treating colds is the yarrow plant. Along with such other herbs as goldenrod and boneset, all of which are available in health food stores and other places that carry herbs, the yarrow is boiled into a tea and drunk periodically.

The point is that many different cultures have produced their own cures for the common cold, and it is obvious that most wouldn't have survived as long as they did if there wasn't something to them.

LET YOUR FINGERS DO THE WALKING
TO CURE A COLD

Here is an acupressure technique that you can use to relieve the congestion and headache typical of a cold. With the padded part of your fingertips, use a moderate amount of pressure and begin first on the middle of your forehead. Using your right index finger on your right side, and your left index finger on your left side, apply pressure all the way down to your nostrils. The pressure should last no more than five seconds in each area. Move your fingers down toward your nostrils in three equal motions; then apply an even pressure on the bridge of your nose, on both sides. Now apply pressure to the lower portions of your nose, in equidistant motions as before.

Next repeat the three equidistant motions in reverse, moving from the eyebrows up to the middle of the forehead, where you started. Apply pressure on both sides at the very top of the head, halfway to the hairline, and at the bottom of the hairline.

It works. Try it.

MARY C.'S STRANGE EXPERIENCE

Vitamin C is known for the vital role it plays in maintaining health, but its specialty is in the prevention of colds. A middle-aged woman, Mary C., was a secretary in New York City. She had to take the bus to work, and during New York's chilly winters she often had a bad cold as a result of waiting at the bus stop. One day she heard from a friend about the effects large doses of Vitamin C have on colds. The next time Mary felt a scratchy throat and a runny nose coming on, she bought a bottle of vitamin C in one-gram tablets, and took one tablet every three hours. Much to her surprise, the early symptoms disappeared by the next day. Now whenever Mary feels the symptoms coming on, she takes vitamin C in large doses; she also takes regular maintenance doses of C in smaller amounts. At last report, she hadn't had a cold in more than a year.

A FEW MORE UNUSUAL REMEDIES
YOU CAN TRY AT HOME

Here are a few miscellaneous cold remedies you should be able to try at home:

Maple Syrup: By the time the first colonists arrived in New England, the Indians had been using maple sugar and its syrup as cold remedies for untold years. The French who settled in Illinois learned of this "exceeding good remedy for colds and rheumatisms" from the Indians in 1771. Almost all of the various tribes knew about the efficacy of maple sugar and syrup in treating colds. If you try this remedy at home, however, make sure you are getting 100% pure maple syrup. Dilute it with a little water and drink it several times a day, hot or cold.

Sarsaparilla: Sarsaparilla, a root, was originally used by the Indians as a cough medicine — the root was pulverized and boiled in water, then consumed as a tea. For many years, sarsaparilla was a key ingredient in root beer. Many health food stores now carry root beer made from real roots, purified water, and honey; sarsaparilla is generally available from herbalists and in health food stores, as are most of the herbs mentioned in this book.

Licorice: Licorice in its different forms has medicinal value for congested throats and lungs, and is particularly helpful in cases of dry, hacking coughs. Licorice contains saponins, natural substances which break up and loosen mucus in the air passages. Licorice cough drops are also available.

Rosemary: A famous cure for colds has been a tea made from the common spice rosemary. The English herbalist Culpepper first noted in the seventeenth century that making a condensed tea of the leaves in wine, and drinking it, would "cure all cold diseases, drowsiness, dumb palsy, falling sickness, lethargy, loss of speech, a stinking breath, or pains in gums and teeth."

Peppermint Oil: Ordinary peppermint oil from the dried leaves of the flowering plant was recommended long ago by the British herbalist Leyel. He said it was an invaluable inhalant for diseased lungs and that it destroyed germs, stopped coughs, diminished phlegm, and increased nutrition and health. In lozenge form, it was said to quickly relieve cold symptoms. It is available in oil form and in cough drops at many drug stores as well as health food stores.

Tarragon: Langham, a sixteenth-century herbalist, recommended the spice tarragon, boiled in water for a few minutes, mixed with honey and drunk as a tea, because it was good for coughing and roughness of the throat. Tarragon is common in all spice sections.

Slippery Elm: The bark of the elm tree known as slippery elm is available in powdered form in both health food stores and drug stores. Slippery elm lozenges as well as cough drops are to be found in both. The bark is used as a poultice by mixing the powder with an equal amount of cornstarch, and adding dark mustard, such as French Dijon available in many grocery stores — not more than 10 per cent. The mixture should be spread on a large square of muslin and applied to the chest overnight. Slippery elm can also be mixed with water and drunk as a tea.

DEBBIE Y.'S VOICE CURE

A singer, Debbie Y., found that due to the hoarseness resulting from a cold, she could hardly sing a note. Her voice teacher recommended that she drink a glass of hot water every hour, in which had been mixed three teaspoons of pure honey and several good squeezes of a fresh lemon. After she had drunk a few glasses of this mixture, her voice returned with all its former strength and even a little extra added resonance. Her throat was no longer scratchy and raw. She now uses this mixture whenever she has to sing for any length of time, whether she has a cold or not.

THE MIRACULOUS EFFECTS OF GINSENG

Much has been written about ginseng and its health-giving properties because so many different cultures have used it for so many thousands of years. Chapter 10 is devoted entirely to the subject. One of the chief uses for ginseng is for colds, and as far back as colonial times its effectiveness in curing them was noted. For example, one colonist wrote, "The Root...is of wonderful Vertue in many Cases, particularly to raise the Spirits and promote Perspiration, which makes it a Specifick in Colds and Coughs.... I carry'd home this Treasure, with as much Joy, as if every Root had been the Graft of the Tree of Life, and wash'd and dry'd it carefully."

Ginseng is available almost everywhere vitamins are sold. The authors have even seen it in liquor stores. It comes in powdered form, as a tea, in capsules, and in many other ways.

LAUGH, DON'T COUGH

Last but not least, don't forget that humor is a potent remedy against all sorts of diseases. Humor was also an important ingredient in many early American cold cures, such as this one:

"Take one tall silk hat, a four-poster bed, and a bottle of brandy. To Be Taken As Follows — Put the tall silk hat on the right-hand post of the foot of the bed, lie down and arrange yourself comfortably, drink the brandy, and when you see a tall silk hat on the right and left bedposts you are cured."

The authors recommend that a good dose of humor be mixed with all the aforementioned cold remedies.

SUMMARY

The common cold is one great puzzle modern science has not been able to solve. Although it has been proven that colds are caused by viruses, science has yet to come up with an anti-cold vaccine or even an effective remedy for the unpleasant side effects. And most people know that there doesn't seem to be any *one* remedy that always cures, although Vitamin C is as close as anyone has come to an all-around cold cure. What is sure is that despite all the television advertising, one should avoid patent medicines. If they do relieve the pains of a cold, they often make up for it by making the cold last longer. Through the centuries, however, people have discovered different remedies can help cope with a cold — and this chapter tells of most of them, from chicken soup and bed rest to garlic, foods that are naturally high in Vitamin C, honey and apple cider, castor oil and turpentine, catnip tea with lemon, maple syrup, sarsaparilla, licorice, rosemary, peppermint oil, tarragon, slippery elm, ginseng, and last but not least, acupressure and humor.

3

THE NATURAL WAY TO PROMOTE HEALTHFUL SLEEP AND ENJOY YOUTHFUL VITALITY

"It's all in the mind," they say about fatigue and insomnia; unfortunately, this is the sad truth, at least to a great extent. This is not to say, of course, that there aren't real physiological causes for fatigue, but nonetheless, our minds will often tell us we are fatigued when our bodies are quite capable of expending more energy. This has been tested in double-blind scientific studies — patients who were given a pill that supposedly contained anti-fatigue properties had less fatigue in performing specific tasks than those who did not receive the placebo.

Fatigue can often result from depression or monotony. It can easily be relieved by a change of scenery or just the thought of doing something you enjoy: consider the way you might feel after a hard day at the office, for instance. You're rather tired, right? Suppose, however, you come home from work feeling dead-tired, and somebody suggests doing something you really enjoy doing. Watch that fatigue disappear as if by magic! So much of fatigue is mental that you yourself often can take it in hand and banish it forever. Isn't that a refreshing thought?

Sometimes the best cure for fatigue is to get more exercise. This may sound paradoxical, but it really isn't. Fatigue can be caused by too little physical activity. Once your body perks up, however, you begin to feel a whole new sense of well-being, and your depression lifts. Depression, fatigue, sluggishness, boredom — they all come in the same dreary package. Exercise, however, can mark that package "Return to Sender!" Sometimes, of course, you might have to force yourself to get out of your comfortable chair and march out the front door. It may seem to be more trouble than it's worth. But once you start to exercise regularly, you will become convinced of the ability of physical activity to eliminate fatigue. Not only will you have far more energy than you thought was possible, but you will also find yourself sleeping better at night, too.

It has been estimated that, of every one hundred people who say they suffer from being constantly fatigued, only twenty percent have an actual physical reason for saying this. Of course, there are physical reasons that we get tired, even if those physical reasons are sometimes first caused by the mental ones. Many of the following remedies are offered in that spirit — these are nature's general tonics. They will in the long run give you something much better than the various synthetic drugs people take for extra energy, drugs which often leave dangerous side effects as well. Throughout the centuries, people on different parts of the globe have discovered natural remedies that give them better endurance, and banish fatigue and its ironically parallel malady, insomnia, as well as improving the whole tone of their lives. These are the natural tonics we will discuss in this chapter. They are important to learn about, because the alternatives that so many people in our high-pressure society use today end up aggravating the situation. That is why so many folks live "on the edge," and are always just inches away from total psychological and physiological breakdowns.

FIRST, WHAT WE SHOULDN'T BE DOING

We know that the country seems to live on coffee and yet more coffee. It's amazing how many of us gulp down 15 to 20 cups of coffee in a day. Most of us would probably blanch if we realized just how close to the lethal four-gallon limit we get with our excessive consumption of caffeine. And it's not only coffee that's loaded with caffeine — tea, for instance, has three-quarters the amount of caffeine instant coffee has, and colas have half the amount. We know how many people are addicted to colas. Our children and teenagers are also becoming caffeine addicts via their chocolate and cocoa consumption, either directly in candy bars, or indirectly in pastries, cereals, and milk. Caffeine is also present in patent medicines, "wake-me up" preparations, or so-called cold and headache remedies made up usually of aspirin and caffeine. The caffeine serves this purpose: If you're a caffeine addict, you start to get headaches when you are running low on caffeine — that's because caffeine is an addictive drug, and you're beginning to suffer withdrawal symptoms. So you take caffeine in a pill to get rid of those symptoms!

In 1974 Dr. John F. Greden, a psychiatrist at the University of Michigan's Medical Center in Ann Arbor, reported in the American Journal of Psychiatry on the side-effects of caffeine addiction. He listed irritability, nervousness, headaches, rapid breathing, insomnia, ringing in the ears, and twitching. Dr. Greden described one woman, a nurse; her doctors, after considerable laboratory analysis, decided she was having a classic "anxiety reaction," because she was suffering many of the reactions described above. They could do nothing for her except prescribe powerful sedatives, so she decided to see if it was something in her own diet. She finally realized it was, because she had recently purchased a new coffee pot which made coffee taste so good that she was drinking more of it than ever before. It was when she drank the coffee that she had the worst symptoms, so she tried an experiment — for 36 hours she didn't drink a single cup of coffee. This completely cured her of the "anxiety syndrome" that the doctors with all their laboratory analysis had not been able to diagnose. Since then, further research has shown that coffee has this bad effect because it destroys thiamine (vitamin B1), which enables your body to properly relax. The moral here should be obvious.

A PEACHY REMEDY

Now of course neither the remedy we are about to tell you about, nor any of the others you'll read about later in this chapter, exclude some kind of mild exercise as part of the anti-fatigue/anti-insomnia "prescription." Walking, swimming, bicycling or other regular exercise will help eliminate both fatigue and insomnia. But as a general tonic, you might want to take a leaf out of the traditional remedies of the old Southwest. An old-fashioned but remarkably effective energizer comes to us from the always-vigorous Southwestern Indians. They wash away fatigue in minutes with a general tonic made from peach leaves. The leaves are steeped in water, and the resulting tea is used both as a remedy for asthma and in cases of fatigue and debility. It is even valued for its effects in regulating menstrual imbalances, when given as a warm douche.

PLANTS THAT INDUCE SLEEP...
IN MINUTES

The Sleep Pillow: Our brave pioneer forebears, the frontier Americans from the 1830s and 1840s, also pioneered some intriguing remedies for getting to sleep. One of their favorites was the "sleep pillow." The feathers usually found in pillows were replaced with some dried hops and pine needles. Another similar remedy was prepared by mixing together in a small cloth bag three ounces of rose petals, two ounces of mint leaves, and half an ounce of powdered cloves. The small bag was then placed under the regular pillow at night.

Peppermint Tea: For many years, herbalists used a tea made from peppermint leaves in the belief that it was equal to coffee or tea when it came to imparting energy. It was also supposed to banish mental depression and induce sleep. Modern herbalists also attribute to peppermint tea the power to banish headaches and indigestion.

Grapes: Over the years, many health-giving properties have been noted for the lowly grape. Sometime back we decided to try the recommendation of an authority who said that grapes are a general topic for the whole system. One day, for what reason we could not immediately tell, both the authors awoke not feeling terribly well. Perhaps the reason we didn't feel well was that we had to go shopping that morning, because we had a dinner guest scheduled for that evening, and neither of us were in a mood for shopping. Shortly after entering the gleaming food emporium, we noticed that the fruit section was full of wonderful grapes, in all their different shades and flavors. Then we remembered the words we had read suggesting that grapes were a tonic. That was enough. Maybe grapes are a tonic merely because they taste so good, but the feeling engendered by them was enough to banish the fatigue that had plagued us early that morning. We went on to have a wonderful day, without a trace of fatigue until just before bedtime. One of the wonderful things about living in California, as we do, is that grapes are available nearly all the time. We are not sure that grapes will banish everyone's fatigue, but they generally do for us; they are indeed a tonic that drives away any feelings of fatigue. The only problem is that they go so fast! Everyone loves to eat them! With grapes, taking your medicine is not a bad thing.

Lettuce: After Hippocrates, the next great figure in ancient medicine was Galen, who claimed that he was relieved of insomnia by eating lettuce. "I had so accustomed myself in my youth to stay awake and study that in age I was much irritated by inability to sleep. Against this annoyance I have found no better remedy than eating lettuce in the evening." Galen didn't mention how much lettuce he ate, but the vegetable has few calories, so eat a good quantity.

A SOOTHING BEVERAGE FOR
BETTER SLEEP

The Journal of Clinical Pharmacology, in its November/December, 1973 issue, reported on twelve hospital patients, all of whom were undergoing cardiac catheterization, which makes sleep rather difficult. Research showed that chamomile tea proved to be invaluable in aiding the patients' sleep; not only were they able to sleep deeply, but they could also be easily awakened by the hospital personnel when the need arose, after which the patients were able to fall asleep again immediately. Chamomile flowers are a very common commodity in health food stores and at herbalists' shops; there are also commercial tea preparations that are easily obtainable.

WHAT'S ALL THE FUSS ABOUT
L-TRYPTOPHAN?

You may have heard about a miraculous "sleep drug" known as L-tryptophan, available in tablet form. But did you also know than L-tryptophan is easily obtained by drinking a glass of warm milk before retiring? The sleep-inducing properties of warm milk are due to the presence of L-tryptophan. L-tryptophan is actually an amino acid (protein component) naturally present in such high protein foods as milk, cheese, eggs and meat. It is also present in some high-carbohydrate foods, such as potatoes and bread. That is why it is a good idea to eat a high-carbohydrate snack half an hour before bedtime. Many high-carbohydrate foods may actually contain more L-tryptophan than protein foods. You may prefer the old familiar glass of warm milk, however. There was a reason mother used to give you cookies and milk before bedtime.

AN 1897 HOUSEHOLD REMEDY
FOR FATIGUE

This is the text of a household remedy against fatigue, which dates from 1897: "When very weak or weak from exhaustion, heat some milk to the scalding point, then sip it as hot as possible. It refreshes almost instantly. How often we hear women who do their own work say that by the time they have prepared a meal and it is ready for the table they are too tired to eat. One way to mitigate this evil is to take, about ½ hour before dinner, a raw egg, beat it light, put in a little sugar, flavor it and drink it down. It will remove the faint, tired out feeling, and will not spoil your appetite for dinner."

MORE OLD-FASHIONED INSOMNIA
REMEDIES

Our pioneer ancestors had interesting ways of dealing with insomnia. For example, one frontier insomnia cure suggested sleeping in a dimly-lit room. The sufferer was to lie with his head propped up, and then was to select an object a little to one side, which he was to look at steadily, until his eyes became "well a-weary, and refreshing sleep will soon follow."

Many of our ancestors apparently knew of the value of the various uses of hot water as a cure for insomnia.

They also knew about rubbing the body and extremities with a brush, a towel, or even with the bare hand. Another remedy that was supposed to be sensational for insomnia was taking cold water, putting it on a cloth, and rubbing it on the nape of the neck. Various herbs and foods were recommended, including the following: "Eat a dish of baked onions or try eating a thick slice of bread and butter, sprinkled with a little cayenne pepper." Wisely, it added the warning not to overdo this last treatment.

We've found new hope for insomnia relief in the form of the kinds of hot beverages we consume before bedtime in our house. They are beverages our highly-esteemed forefathers imbibed, with such good results. We have used with success hot lemonade and hot ginger tea. Another one we've used on only a couple of occasions, but with equal success. This was when we were trying to get to sleep with a headache. We mixed the juice of a lemon with oil of roses and applied it to the forehead. Next time one of us gets a headache just before going to sleep, we are going to try another old remedy we read of a while ago. This calls for washing "the head in a decoction of dill seeds and smell(ing) of it frequently."

THE REST-INDUCTING PROPERTIES
OF LIGHT

Light has many health benefits, which may be part of the reason so many folks left the places they originally hailed from and moved to our home state of California. Living out-of-doors as we do, even in the winter months, we Californians are probably luckier than the rest of the states. It has really been only in the last century or so that people have lived more and more indoors, out of the sunlight. You know, of course, that the sun makes vitamin D in our systems when it hits our skins. Some scientists have argued that fluorescent lighting is not a very healthful thing. We believe if you want to feel fully rested, and restore your energy, and eliminate chronic fatigue, get out of the fluorescent light used in office buildings. Spend more time out of the incadescent-lighted homes we all live in. Throw open your windows to the birds and the sunlight outside whenever you can. Or better yet, just go out of doors and let the sunlight bathe you in its glorious rays!

SOMETHING TO THINK ABOUT
WHILE COUNTING SHEEP

You may actually be getting much more sleep than you think you've been getting. We've noticed this about each other. When one of us complains he or she didn't get much sleep, the other, who really did spend most of the night up working on a project, observed that actually the supposed insomnia victim was asleep most of the time. There are many gray areas in sleep, points at which we aren't exactly awake, or completely asleep, either. It may be more a question of quality than quantity. But in any event, take relief from the fact that your insomnia might well not be half as bad as you think it is.

SPICE RACK REMEDIES

When it comes to fatigue, you might need to look no farther than your kitchen spice rack to find effective remedies. For instance, sage was used by the Dutch as a preventative of illness and for the rejuvenation of "eyes, brains and glands." Some herbalists use it to cure insomnia, while other herbalists believe it deals well with lethargy and fatigue. Sage leaves can be dried and boiled, then drunk as a tea; and the powdered spice can also be added in generous amounts to spicy foods. The Dutch used to eat it in handfuls as a snack.

Summer savory was also known as a powerful remedy. The great English herbalist Langham first wrote about it, saying that savory was good "against lethargy or drowsiness," and that it "did quickeneth the wits or braine."

FATIGUE FROM FEAR OF LIFE

Fatigue can result from being overwhelmed by life, but it can also be reversed. When James Boswell wrote his famous biography of Samuel Johnson, he described how, every time Johnson had a task to perform, Johnson would become so tired that he would be unable to face the work at hand. He couldn't even figure out what time it was on the clock. Charles Darwin, the great scientist, would become seriously ill and fatigued at the thought of making a public appearance or beginning a journey. The testimony of other creative men and women, however, is that once they get going, the work at hand is rarely as bad as the thought of it. By resolutely attacking the work at hand, one can banish the fatigue and malaise that go with putting it off.

BART E.'S SURE-FIRE INSOMNIA REMEDY

We close this chapter with a couple of interesting home remedies for insomnia. One was discovered by Bart E., who could never get to sleep at night. He found, however, that if he took a large onion, put it in a good-sized container, poured boiling water over it, then steeped, stirred, strained and drank the resulting liquid, he could sleep like a baby all night long.

Another insomnia remedy: Mix two teaspoons of cooked oatmeal in a glassful of cold milk, and add a teaspoon of honey. Drink it down, then follow it with a glass of hot milk.

SUMMARY

There is nothing more wonderful than a good night's sleep after a hard day. If you've been doing hard physical work all day and just before you get into bed you begin to realize just how fatigued you are, that is very natural — and good. If the sleep is good, you wake up the next morning refreshed and ready to go. And you don't get fatigued easily. This is, of course, the ideal state; and it isn't what always happens to us. Sometimes, though we sleep, we wake up, still fatigued. And even after being fatigued all day, we still can't get a good night's sleep.

The truth is that a great deal of the fatigue and sleep problems that plague human beings are in the head. This means that to some extent they are the products of our own imaginations. But our imaginations also depend on the health of our bodies — and oftentimes there are remedies that will correct something that's out of balance in the body. So we feel better; and the world seems to be a better place.

This chapter has recommended a number of remedies to try. And things to avoid as you begin to win the battle to banish fatigue and regain the ability to have a good night's sleep again.

4

CONQUERING CONSTIPATION, DIARRHEA, AND INDIGESTION

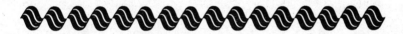

Anyone who has ever suffered from constipation, indigestion, or diarrhea — and who hasn't? — knows that sometimes our poor, tired bodies seem to be nothing more than a mass of plumbing. And as with all plumbing, there are times when it doesn't work properly. To make matters worse, ours is not like the plumbing found in mechanical contrivances like cars or airplanes; our system does not contain any replaceable parts — at least not yet. Our plumbing may be repairable, but it isn't made up of interchangeable pieces. Perhaps worst of all, our personal plumbing is very affected by the state of our nerves, often in what seem to be strange and arbitrary ways. The result of this is all too often pain — sometimes excruciating pain.

THE ALMOST UNIVERSAL PROBLEM

The most universal problem of all, because it is the most common and often the hardest to cure, is constipa-

71

tion. It can have many causes, some physical, some mental. Digestion is often disrupted by a nervous state, and there is no doubt that many people are obsessed with the notion of what they perceive to be "correct" elimination. But there is no such thing as a medical need for "regularity." Often the delineation is rather thin between "regularity" and "irregularity," but ultimately there is no hard-and-fast rule as to how often a person should visit the toilet. The daily bowel movement which has been highly touted over the years is an exaggerated notion pushed by the manufacturers of various laxatives. A natural elimination pattern depends on a number of factors — an individual's diet, mental state, and the state of his bowels.

WHY "HOLDING IT" IS BAD

It is a sad commentary on our modern society that we often "psych" ourselves into a perpetual state of constipation. People who grow up with too many family members and not enough bathrooms, for instance, almost invariably develop the bad habit of "holding it," which causes chronic constipation that can last a lifetime if the bad habit is not unlearned at some point. And our diet is so lacking in the roughage needed for clean, complete evacuation of the bowel that many of us are obliged to turn to harsh laxatives for relief. An improved intake of fresh fruits, vegetables and whole grains would not only solve the constipation, but would greatly improve our nutrition as well. Stress, too, plays a big part in causing constipation. We will examine these factors in greater detail.

THE ROLE OF NERVES
IN CONSTIPATION

If our digestive and eliminative systems were simply mechanical, solutions to such problems as constipation, diarrhea, and indigestion would be easily obtained. But when you consider that a relatively large part of the brain is used merely to oversee digestive functions, you can see how interrelated the mental and the physical are when it comes to digestion and elimination.

The nerves introduce another complex element to the entire process. No one knows why exactly, but when people are constipated, they often develop a number of other related symptoms — loss of appetite, exhaustion, dizziness, irritability, bloating, belching, and headaches. Some years ago, a large medical clinic attempted an experiment. Cotton was used to plug the rectums of a number of patients, in order to stimulate a constipated state. When the cotton was removed, the patients' nervousness, irritability, and other side effects vanished as if by magic! It is no wonder, then, that Americans spend nearly half a billion dollars a year on laxatives.

BEWARE THE "BLESSED RELIEF"
THAT COMES IN A BOX!

The FDA says that two per cent of the population takes some sort of laxative every day to aid in elimination. Many people, it is interesting to note, take laxatives not because of direct constipation, but because they feel they must go "regularly." But laxatives do not correct con-

73

stipation; they cause it. After taking a laxative daily for a week or two, a constipation sufferer will discover that he is starting to build up a "tolerance." That is, the natural peristaltic action that normally occurs in the healthy bowel cannot transpire any longer without the aid of the laxative. After the laxative-taking continues for another week or two, the bowel may become so acclimated to the laxative that it will not respond at all without enormous doses. So then the sufferer may attempt to use an enema, which not only purges the bowel of its contents and much of its moisture, but can also severely irritate and inflame the intestinal lining. Then, it's back to the laxative again, until it's time for another enema. Many people follow this foolish cycle over and over again for years.

DIETARY SOLUTIONS FOR
BETTER ELIMINATION

It has been suggested that over half the adult population in this country has some problem with constipation. The reason for this is our modern life style. Stress, a poor diet, and the medications we take routinely are all guilty of causing constipation. Such all-purpose drugs as analgesics, antacids, sedatives, tranquilizers, muscle relaxants, and cough medicines containing codeine contribute materially to elimination difficulties.

Not that early man was free of constipation, though. The Egyptians had numerous constipation cures. In early Greece, Hippocrates, the "father of medicine," warned against the then-current practice of using harsh solutions to empty the bowels — a treatment that was standard in those days for many different ailments. Today, however, constipation has reached epidemic proportions, and the chief culprit is our diet.

The foods we eat bear increasingly little similarity to the original materials from which they are made. Food is endlessly refined, denatured, stripped of vitamins, minerals, and bulk. But we don't need to depend on supermarket hucksters when it comes to filling our shopping carts. If we load up on whole fruits and vegetables, we can lick constipation. Far better than any laxative is a dish of stewed rhubarb, or prunes, plums, and figs. Raw vegetables or fruit, eaten plain or in salads, work wonders with a sluggish bowel. Whole grains, in breads and cereals, are necessary to promote clean evacuations; bran, of course, is an old standby. Natural honey, blackstrap or unsulphured molasses, or olive oil — indeed, any vegetable oil — can also be enormously helpful.

HOW TO EXERCISE YOUR DIGESTIVE SYSTEM FOR NATURAL RELIEF

Exercise is another important factor in curing constipation. Next to eating good food, there is nothing better you can do for relief from constipation than to take a daily walk. It can be short, but it should be brisk. The bowel is, after all, a muscle, and muscles can lose their tone. It is also important to drink enough water and other liquids — you should take as many as eight large glasses a day.

One of the authors has had a terrible problem with constipation for years; she has a very irritable bowel. She can't, for example, stomach any kind of salad dressing or condiment like mayonnaise or mustard. Thus she rarely eats salad, although she does eat attractively prepared vegetables on occasion. Because of insufficient roughage, she was having a terrible problem with constipation. So she began taking a daily walk, in Griffith Park, which happens to be near the authors' home in Los Angeles. Our normal walk was to begin at the bottom of the mountain just below Griffith Park Observatory, and climb to the top, near Dante's View, where Hollywood is spread out below. The walk is about five miles, and much of it is quite rugged and uphill. But don't you say that you can't do this because you are too old. Invariably half of the people climbing that mountain in Griffith Park are in their 60s, and some are in their 80s. They just go marching up that hill, happy, healthy and strong. The walking regimen did wonders, not only for her constipation, but also for insomnia and sluggishness. She knows this because during the rainy seasons (which do, despite popular rumor, plague Los Angeles from time to time) the walking in Griffith Park stops. Then the old problems with constipation invariably return.

SOME FACTS ABOUT INDIGESTION AND DIARRHEA

Indigestion and diarrhea are related problems. Indigestion can be caused by many factors — anything from a case of nerves to bad food habits to actual disease. Sometimes indigestion can be cured by such simple methods as chewing your food slowly and carefully. Diarrhea can often be cured by eliminating excess fruits and vegetables from the diet.

But often, as we have seen, the solution to digestion problem is no one simple thing. Digestion is a complex process. Many remedies have been tried over the ages to improve digestion and elimination, and we will present some of these.

A SURPRISING TIP FOR
BETTER ELIMINATION

The time when the bowel is likely to be most active is between five and seven a.m. If you are a late sleeper, this can throw the whole process off. The body works on something of a diurnal schedule — this is true even of "night owls" — and if you cooperate with it, rather than working against it, you will be much happier in the long run. Set aside a regular time of the morning for elimination. When that time comes, whether you feel "the call" or not, go into the bathroom, sit down, and relax. This may seem overly regimented, but it is aimed toward eradicating the "irritable bowel" syndrome. If you find you cannot pass stool or feel no need to, don't worry about it; try again tomorrow. After a week or two of this process, you will find that you may not have a daily bowel movement, but you will be in far better "tune" with your digestive and eliminative system. Just remember not to strain or rush yourself when the time comes.

Dry stool can be another problem. If you find that you have trouble passing dry stools, check over what medications you are taking. Are you taking diuretics, medication for high blood-pressure, or other water-eliminating drugs? If so, increase your intake of liquids. Or add a couple of teaspoons of pure olive oil to your diet.

77

WHAT YOU CAN LEARN FROM YOUR CAT

Everyone knows that cats are finicky eaters. They have sensitive stomachs and intestines, and are frequently prone to digestive upsets. Most cats, however, like catnip. Maybe we can learn something from our finicky, gourmet felines — for catnip, in the form of catnip tea, has been used to cure upset stomach and digestive problems for hundreds of years.

Catnip's history as a medicinal herb goes back many centuries. The American Indians were the first to use it, and the early settlers quickly learned of its use in treating maladies from upset stomach to colds and even "persistent coughs and hiccups."

Catnip tea should be made up of parts of the whole plant — all the parts that grow above the ground. It should not be boiled, but rather steeped (soaked in hot water) in a covered vessel, like a teapot. It is wise not to take too much catnip tea at one time, since large amounts can cause nausea.

WHAT COLUMBUS DISCOVERED
BESIDES AMERICA

Christopher Columbus not only discovered America, he also stumbled across a fruit remedy used by the natives of the Caribbean to relieve gastric problems resulting from overeating. During his sojourn in the Caribbean, Columbus noticed that if the natives stuffed themselves too much, they were able to avoid unpleasant side effects by eating papaya for dessert. Other sea captains also found that when their sailors ate papaya, the fruit kept their digestive systems healthy.

Papaya contains the powerful enzyme papain, which resembles two digestive enzymes already found in the human stomach — pepsin and trypsin. The best source of papain is the milky juice of the half-ripe fruit. Papain is particularly adept at aiding in the digestion of sometimes hard-to-digest proteins. In fact, meat tenderizers are usually made from unripe papaya. The fruit is becoming increasingly available in supermarkets across the country. Papain is available in health food stores in powder and tablet form.

THE SICILIAN COLIC CURE

Maria D., an Italian-American woman who lived in New England, reported an unusual and rather simple cure for colic in her son. The child was two months old when he developed a terrible case of colic. He cried all night, exhausting everyone in the house. Nothing the doctor gave him seemed to help. Then Maria's mother came up with a solution. She gave the baby a bottle full of what appeared to be water. After he drank it, his colic was quickly released and he never suffered from the problem thereafter.

The bottle contained an old Sicilian cure: Maria's mother had boiled a cup of water with part of a bay leaf for fifteen minutes. The mixture was allowed to cool, then poured into the bottle. Part of the bay leaf — less than half — was the right size dose for the baby; adults, said Maria's mother, could try as many as three whole leaves to get rid of indigestion. The remedy was from the old country and had been in Maria's mother's family for generations.

79

NEW USES FOR AN AGE-OLD REMEDY

A young Mexican doctor, Jose C., was entertaining an English medical colleague in a Mexico City restaurant. The Englishman was amazed that his host could down such an incredible amount of hot sauces without even a hint of stomach distress. How did he do it? Jose smiled. His secret was nothing spectacular. He merely took a teaspoon of olive oil before going out to dinner. "It protects my stomach," he explained.

There's nothing new about the use of olive oil for stomach problems. In the *Encyclopedia of Health and Home*, published in 1921, the oil, taken internally, was said to be useful in inflammation of the stomach and bowels. The recommended dose as a laxative was one tablespoonful; for some patients, it was suggested, even more might be needed. Since olive oil is such a mild remedy, the Encyclopedia pointed out, it should always be used in cases of childhood constipation, rather than harsher remedies such as castor oil.

A CONDIMENT THAT AIDS YOUR STOMACH

Coriander seeds are a common condiment in many parts of the country; the seeds are used in the Southwest and California as a main ingredient in sauces. The use of coriander seeds to aid in stomach problems dates back to before the time of the Spanish conquistadors. A history of plants published in London in 1578 describes how the British used coriander seeds. The seeds "prepared, and taken alone (or covered in Sugar) after meales, closeth up the mouth of the stomache, stayeth vomitting, and helpeth digestion," said the book. At first try chewing up a few of the seeds after eating a meal. If stomach troubles persist, increase the amount slightly.

THE SECRET LIFE OF CHARCOAL

Charcoal has long been used by man in various purifying and cleaning functions. It can also be used in a similar way inside our bodies; particularly for stomach and bowel problems. Many drugstores carry charcoal for medicinal purposes, although it is best to make sure that the charcoal is as fresh as possible, and is made from willow, pine or other such soft woods. Charcoal made from cocoanut shells is also fine. A heaping teaspoon of charcoal should be taken after each and every meal. The charcoal should be placed in a cup, and enough hot water added to make a paste. A dab or two of olive oil should also be included. The mixture should then be drunk at once. Charcoal will absorb many times its own volume in gases in your stomach, and thus is an excellent remedy for excess stomach acid, fermentation, heartburn, and acid dyspepsia.

TWO GREEN REMEDIES FOR
STOMACH TROUBLES

Early European folklorists recommended both cabbage and lettuce for stomach problems. In many parts of Europe today, naturalists continue to prescribe these vegetables for the same purposes. Usually they suggest only slightly cooking the cabbage. Do not use salt. Also, do not use vegetables that have been cooked for too long a time or cooked twice, for this lessens their effectiveness as a stomach remedy. Another side benefit, according to one of the early European pioneers of these remedies: "Eaten at the end of a meal they remove all the effects of drinking too much wine."

THE AMAZING PROPERTIES
OF CARAWAY SEEDS

Next time you bite down on some rye bread with caraway seeds, do so with respect. Those little seeds do a lot more besides making bread taste better. Anne Boleyn changed the course of English history with them. As everyone knows, Henry VIII was overly fond of food and drink, as his passions for seven-hour-long feasts amply demonstrated. Henry's royal physicians stood by at these events in order to help their monarch survive his bacchanalia; apparently His Majesty was much troubled with indigestion and other stomach troubles — not very surprising when you consider the vast amounts of food he was capable of putting away.

The comely Anne Boleyn filled her pillbox with caraway seeds and managed to find a seat near the king. When the great man began hiccuping, she pulled out her pillbox and offered him a handful. To his amazement, the little seeds kept his indigestion at bay. The rest, as they say, was history — although history dealt more kindly with Henry, indigestion and all, than it did with the lovely but doomed Anne Boleyn.

Not surprisingly, caraway seeds found their way into the writings of various English herbalists, such as Culpepper, who lived about a century after Henry VIII ate his last banquet. Culpepper described caraway seeds as "a most admirable remedy for those that are troubled with wind or overeating." He also suggested that the roots as well as the seeds of the caraway be taken for gastric problems.

The tradition is carried on when the seeds are used in cooking nowadays. But caraway's history as an aid to healthy digestion goes back to the Greeks and Romans. Julius Caesar was a great believer in caraway, and in the Persian Empire during the sixth century, caraway seeds were considered so valuable that they were used as a medium of exchange.

The entire plant was sometimes eaten, but it was more typical to take the seeds and make a tea of them. Another method that might be interesting, and is very much a traditional way of using caraway seeds for their medicinal effect, is to fry the seeds and put them on a hot cloth over the belly to quell "pains of wind and colic." You might also dip the seeds in sugar, after they have been moistened or buttered, and eat half a spoonful before breakfast and after each of the rest of the day's meals.

THE CASE FOR GINGER ROOT

Ginger root is used in both Japanese and Chinese cooking, and has long had a reputation as a digestive aid in the West, although it hasn't become a standard ingredient in many other cuisines. Nonetheless, as we have studied herbs, we have found recommendations for ginger root as an aid to digestion in books going back as far as the sixteenth century and in books as recent as last week. Apparently what ginger can do, especially if you take it in the form of a syrup, is stimulate stomach secretion and relieve gas distention. The Germans usually drink powdered ginger root as a tea. Dried or ground ginger is boiled with water and red wine, and the resulting tea is taken not only for stomach cramps, indigestion, and colic, but for colds and fever as well.

A REMEDY THAT WAS WORTH A "MINT"

Bernice S., a woman from the Midwest, was visiting her sister, who was recuperating from a gallbladder operation and was in constant pain. The pain was due, not to the operation, but to the gas pains that had resulted from it. Bernice had brought with her some dried mint leaves from her garden, and knowing that mint had a reputation for curing stomach problems, she brewed some mint tea for her sister. The remedy worked right away, and Bernice's sister never had another attack of gas.

Mint leaves are a very common commodity in most parts of the country. They are available dried, as an herb, or in the form of mint teas, which can be purchased at almost any grocery store. Or you can grow your own plants. Mint and its leaves can be chewed whole, prepared as a tea, or added to cold drinks such as lemonade.

FOLK REMEDIES FOR CONSTIPATION
AND DIARRHEA

Americans in the last century had a variety of remedies for constipation, including the following:

1. Take a newly-laid hen's egg, add three times its bulk in water, beat it for thirty minutes, and take in the morning on an empty stomach; then once or twice in the day. Do so for a week or so, and this will "strengthen the system."

2. Stew figs in olive oil until plump and tender, add honey and lemon juice, boil until thick, and consume.

3. Make a strong tea from the leaves and blossoms of the peach tree, then take a teaspoonful every hour; or make a syrup for stronger effect, made by boiling the juice slowly with honey or molasses.

These are early American diarrhea remedies:

1. Burn cork until it is completely charred. Reduce it to a power and mix with an equal amount of sugar, a teaspoon of brandy, a little grated nutmeg, a teaspoon of essence of peppermint, and a tablespoon or two of water. Take as needed, a teaspoon or two at a time.

2. Mix a tablespoon of vinegar and a teaspoon of fine salt in a wineglass full of warm water. Drink every half hour until relief is forthcoming.

AN OLD PIONEER'S REMEDY

According to P.F. Bowker, an old pioneer, the best preventative of stomach disorders was refined chalk, which, of course, is lime. His remedy called for first getting some peach leaves, or bark from the roots of black cherry trees, which is pounded into a fine powder. Then that powder is mixed with an equal quantity of chalk in a glass of hot water, to be sipped after each meal. Bowker claimed that this remedy never failed him.

A COMMON FOOD THAT CAN CURE DIARRHEA

Those who suffer from diarrhea would be well advised to eat rice. A cup of rice boiled in eight cups of water or milk for an hour will aid tremendously in cases of obstinate or long-standing diarrhea. Needless to say, people suffering from constipation should cut down on their rice intake.

MISCELLANEOUS METHODS
FOR AIDING DIGESTIVE ILLS

Here are some various concoctions that people have used over the years to obtain relief for their digestive ills.

Agrimony and burdock are both good for any type of digestive disorder. They are readily available from health food stores and some drug stores in capsules, powdered, and dried form. Take five grams of agrimony three times a day. Use a teaspoon of burdock to a cup of boiling water and steep for ten minutes; drink three times daily.

A teaspoon of dill seeds boiled in a cup of water for fifteen minutes, then strained and slowly sipped, will help to calm an irritable stomach. Mustard seeds are also good as a remedy for gastritis. Swallow one seed with a little water the first day, two the second, three the next, and keep adding a seed every day until finally twenty seeds a day are being consumed. Then reverse the process, subtracting a seed every day until you are finally back to one. The seeds should be washed down with water the first thing in the morning while your stomach is still empty.

Parsley tea is said to be good for stomach cramps — a teaspoon of parsley leaves to a cup of boiling water, steeped for five minutes. Drink as needed.

Our friend L. John Harris, America's garlic king, also suggests that for a stomachache, slice garlic into yogurt. Leave standing for several hours before eating, he advises. He also adds that you can remove the garlic before eating the mixture if you do not like the taste or effects of raw garlic. In other words, simply eat the garlified yogurt, but without the garlic. That, he insists, will do the trick for a bum stomach. The reason is that garlic neutralizes the bacteria that are bad for your stomach.

SUMMARY

Some people have iron stomachs, it seems. They can eat anything and never do their stomachs get upset. But these lucky souls are in a minority — most of us know of foods that will upset our stomachs. Many of us have stomachs that are constantly upset. Furthermore, digestion is obviously connected with elimination, and everyone knows of the miseries that can be involved at that end as well.Worse yet, the whole digestive and eliminative process is connected to our entire nervous system — the one affects the other. If you feel jittery, your stomach and bowels will reflect that. Luckily, however, there are many natural remedies that can greatly improve both your digestive and eliminative systems. Chapter 6 also contains constipation remedies.

5

NEW HELP FOR HEADACHES

Most people are all too familiar with the agonizing pain of headaches. The worst thing about headaches, though, is that there seems to be little you can do to relieve them except reach for the aspirin bottle. But there are alternatives to aspirin, which at best will only cover the symptoms of the problem, and at worst will do considerable damage to your stomach lining. In this chapter you will discover what the alternatives are, and how you can use them to banish headaches.

When you get a headache, what your body is doing is sending a signal to your brain, warning that something is wrong somewhere. The basic cause of the pain is a change in the flow of the blood, but this is not to be confused with blood pressure. Changes in blood flow can be caused by a wide variety of things, but the end result is always a diminished blood flow, and hence a lesser amount of oxygen, with the final result being a terrible headache.

WHY WE GET HEADACHES

A large number of the causes of headaches are not easy to control. Many of our headaches come from our environment — and short of changing that environment, there isn't a lot that can be done. For example, people in the black ghettoes, for example, suffer a higher incidence of headaches brought on by depression than do other segments of the society. Modern urban environments thrust all kinds of unnatural situations on us, and one of the results of coping with these situations is the splitting headache. Medications, such as antibiotics, can also be a culprit, along with a variety of other causes, including stress, fatigue, or an argument with one's spouse. Some people develop headaches after eating certain foods — alcohol, cheese, chocolate, and citrus fruits are the main examples of these.

Stress and tension are probably the parents of most headaches, although it is interesting to note that tense headaches usually occur toward the end of the stressful period, when the stress is beginning to subside. Fatigue and hunger can also bring on headaches. People tend to experience these headaches at the end of the day without knowing why. Eyestrain can also cause headaches, and sinus headaches are almost always triggered by changes in the air pressure outside. Infections also cause headaches.

TRY A NAP OR A SNACK

Often the cause of a headache is simply a missed meal. Other times a nap is the cure. Sleep therapy has been used quite successfully in headache clinics — when the patient feels a headache coming on, he is given something to make him sleep, and often awakes without pain.

It must also be said that an aspirin is not the best way to deal with a headache for other reasons. As we already said, the headache is a way your body has of telling you something. Recurrent headaches can sometimes indicate a more serious illness. It is estimated that even in cases of painful recurrent headaches, barely two percent are attributable to organic causes.

WATCH THAT ICE CREAM

If you are addicted to ice cream — and many of us certainly fall into that category — you'll be amazed to know that some of those sharp but short headaches you're been suffering from are the result of your addiction. This is because headaches are sometimes caused by cold. For example, if it is a hot day, and you go inside to a cold air-conditioned building, that too can cause a headache.

MIGRAINES AND "CLUSTER" HEADACHES

The best-known of the really disabling headaches are migraines, and it has been estimated that up to twenty per cent of the population suffers from them — usually far more women than men. Interestingly enough, when women migraine sufferers become pregnant, they don't suffer from migraines during their pregnancies, although the headaches reoccur after the pregnancy ends. Men suffer more than women from "cluster" headaches, which sometimes have associations with heart disease or ulcers. Alcohol should particularly be avoided, because it exacerbates this problem — even shaving lotion should be avoided.

FOODS THAT CAUSE HEADACHES

Many people have food allergies that result in headaches. You can obviously experiment with yourself to see if you are a victim of any food allergies, and then take appropriate action. The most famous of these is the "Chinese restaurant syndrome," which refers to a peculiarly painful headache (and sometimes faceache as well) caused by the large amounts of monosodium glutamate often used in the cooking. Other chemical additives in foods can also have a similar reaction — so if you notice a link between a headache and a particular food you just ate, read the contents carefully and you might find what's been causing that headache. But some people are also sensitive to particular amino acids that are found in cheese, nuts, pork, and fish. And alcoholic beverages are frequent headache producers; red wine has often brought on some real doozies, and mixed drinks seem to cause more morning-after agony than taking your alcohol straight.

DIGITAL RELIEF

One massage technique we have used with success is the following: Find the base of your skull behind your ears and then trace it down, toward the spine. On each side of the point where your spine connects into the base of the skull, you'll find a slight depression. Apply pressure with a rotary motion of your thumb to this area. Massage the entire area. Let your mouth drop open to relax your jaws.

HOPS FOR HEADACHES

Some years back, a Canadian doctor claimed to have cured patients suffering from nervous headache by having them drink a tea made from hops. The patients were directed to drink a small cupful every three hours, or every two hours if the patient was having an especially hard time. The remedy produced results in a day or two.

HOW AN HERBAL MIXTURE CURED
JANE L.'S HEADACHE

Jane L., a young woman, had suffered from migraine headaches for nearly ten years. She finally obtained permanent relief with an herbal remedy composed of two ounces of wood betony (frequently used in headache remedies), an ounce of rosemary, and an ounce of skullcap. The mixture was added to a pint of cold water, brought to a boil, simmered for two minutes, strained, and then left to cool. A wineglass full of this liquid three times daily completely cured Jane L. within days of her long-standing affliction. Another traditional herbal remedy — this one from the Ozarks — is to consume wild peppermint.

THE TRADITIONAL HEADACHE REMEDY

The common herb rosemary has been used to cure headaches for centuries. Young monks used to collect the tops of rosemary bushes, which were mixed with the plant's leaves and flowers and brewed as a tea for curing headaches. The herb acquired an early reputation for being able to cure all sorts of head ailments. Culpepper, the well-known early English herbalist, recommended "a strong decoction of the leaves in Wine" for curing "dullness of the mind, stupidness, a weak memory, or the usual giddiness in wives." The Romans thought of rosemary as a "fine brain tonic." Herbalists frequently recommend it not only for headaches, but as a cure for nervousness, insomnia, and even colds. A popular folk remedy suggests holding a small bottle of spirits of rosemary to the nose and inhaling the fumes, as well as rubbing the liquid on the temples, forehead, veins to the neck, and behind the ears; it is supposed to make a headache simply vanish.

SEVERAL UNUSUAL OLD-FASHIONED HEADACHE CURES

Our pioneer ancestors had to deal with many health problems. They found unusual and effective ways to eliminate problems like headaches, which they suffered from just as modern folks do.

The Potato Cure: One headache cure was to peel and slice raw potatoes and then bind them on the forehead in a cloth that reached around the neck.

The Mustard Poultice: Yet another remedy that was effective was to make a poultice of ground mustard seed, then apply it to the back of the neck between the shoulders.

Monroe's Foot Cure: In 1824, John Monroe, writing in the *American Botanist and Family Physician*, suggested taking the fresh leaves of common burdock, "fresh roots of a poke," fresh garlic, garden onions, wild onions, or mustard seed, and applying any of them to the soles of the feet. This, he said, was a very effective cure for many kinds of headaches.

The Lemon Cure: For periodical morning headaches, the sufferer is directed to take a thin piece of fresh lemon peel which has just been freed from the soft, fibrous part of the fruit, and place it on each of the temples before the volatile oil evaporates.

The Grape Cure: One traditional remedy calls for using grape leaves, which are beaten and mixed with porridge, such as cooked oatmeal, to make a poultice that is then applied to the forehead.

A Bubbling Remedy: An effective remedy combines half a teaspoon of fresh lemon juice with eight ounces of water, at a temperature that is as warm as it can be and still be comfortably imbibed. A teaspoon of baking soda is then added to this mixture, and it is drunk while the liquid is still bubbling.

Ground Ivy: For quick headache relief, simply take the fresh juice from ground ivy and stuff it up the nose.

Lettuce Compress: Lettuce boiled with oil of rose and used as a compress is especially good for an obstinate headache. Cabbage is also one of the oldest headache cures, including headaches resulting from hangovers, as noted below. But herbalists are split on the best way to take it — some believe it is more effective when cooked until soft. Others maintain it is most effective when eaten raw. We always eat our cabbage raw when we want to get rid of headaches.

Cure for the Headache with Nausea: When you have a headache that is accompanied by nausea, cut four slices of fresh cucumber into a bowl. Add a tablespoon of dried seaweed, and then put in just enough water to cover everything, but no more. Allow the mixture to stand overnight and drink it the first thing in the morning when you wake up.

SUGGESTIONS THAT MIGHT BE WORTH A "MINT" TO HEADACHE SUFFERERS

An old traditional headache cure from Mexico is to paste a fresh mint leaf on the part of the head where the pain is most pronounced. In the United States, a traditional remedy called for simply eating the mint leaf. Despite the different ways in which the plant is used, it certainly says something that traditions from two different countries use the same plant. The early English herbalist Langham recommended that the juice of mint leaves should be dropped into the ears to cure headaches as well as earaches and some forms of deafness.

THE REMEDY THAT CAN'T BE BEET — BUT IS

The pioneer English herbalist Culpepper, as well as his colleague Langham, both recommended beets for curing headaches. "The juice of the barke of the roote" should be squeezed into the nose for migraines and other headaches, Langham said. The use of beets for headaches was also known in the New World, before people like Culpepper and Langham even knew there was a New World. The Navajos had been eating beet roots and applying them topically to cure headaches for generations. Modern herbalists in the Ozarks get their best results with beets against headaches by wilting beet leaves and binding them to the forehead.

TREATMENT WITH HANDS AND FEET

Next time you have a headache, try massaging your feet, or better yet, have someone else do it for you — that will definitely improve the method's effectiveness. Simply rub and knead the feet, and even the ankles and calves, for half an hour. Pay special attention to the fleshy underpart of the big toes, and work around each digit, seeking out the parts that protrude the most. Also couple this method with plunging your hands into water as hot as you can stand it. This has proven to be an effective headache cure for many, many people.

THE UNUSUAL CAUSE OF KAY J.'S
HEADACHE — AND ITS CURE

Kay J., a secretary, often suffered from headaches, but when she went to the doctor seeking relief, no specific organic cause could be found for the headaches. Her physician took an inventory of all Kay's symptoms and decided that hers was a cause of artificial overproduction of positive ions, which were being generated because Kay spent a good deal of time in sealed buildings with climate control. Weather changes can also be responsible for this problem; positive-ion winds plague the populations of Jerusalem and Los Angeles, for instance. Kay's doctor realized what her problem was when she told him that her headaches always lessened in places where there were negative ions, such as beside the crashing surf at the beach, or in the shower at home. Eventually Kay obtained low-cost negative ion generators — one she used on her desk at work and the other at home. These devices cured her headaches. If you live in an area such as Los Angeles, where positive-ion winds blow frequently, and you suffer from frequent headaches and irritability, you might look into these negative-ion generators as a possible solution to your problem.

CURED MEATS AND A CURED HEADACHE

Marshall L. was a fellow who sometimes suffered from severe headaches about half an hour after meals. At first, neither Marshall nor his doctor could figure out the cause, but finally it was discovered that the villain was sodium nitrite, the controversial chemical used by meat processors to improve the esthetic appearance of their products. (Sodium nitrite has also been linked to human cancer in recent studies). Marshall's doctor was obliged to tell his patient that there was, unfortunately, no cure for his nitrite-induced headaches; he simply had to give up cured meats, like ham and bacon. When he did, he no longer suffered from postprandial headaches.

THE DANGERS OF CHEWING GUM

Michael P., a 44-year-old man, was suffering from recurrent bilateral headaches in the frontal and temporal regions. Extensive hospital tests revealed nothing, and Michael was out a lot of money. Then one doctor noticed that Michael had a pronounced tendency towards teeth-grinding, and he asked Michael how much gum he chewed. Michael replied that he had been chewing two or three packs a day for many years. The doctor suggested that he stop chewing gum for a while, and Michael found that, after a week of gumlessness, his headaches were a thing of the past. Periodic checks after this assured that his cure remained effective. It did. Michael has not chewed gum since then.

OF HANGOVERS, HEADACHES, AND OTHER HUMBUGS

Hangovers, which almost always include perfectly horrible headaches, have both physical and psychological causes. For example, if you happen to get quite drunk at the office party and call your boss a buffoon, you'll probably wake up the next morning with a tension headache — the kind that isn't directly caused by alcohol, only indirectly so. The alcohol only served to lower your inhibitions to the point where your "secret self" took over — and you did the rest.

For some people, a hangover may be a symptom of mild withdrawal — alcohol, after all, is addictive. "The morning after" finds your body craving more liquor. It is probably due to this withdrawal that the age-old "hair of the dog that bit you" morning-after cure got started. Oddly enough, this theory has some scientific basis. Another drink taken the morning after an elbow-bending spree can anesthetize you against the powerful stomach discomfort caused by your previous alcohol intake.

Fatigue, depression, diarrhea, nausea, and upset stomach are some of the classic characteristics of hangovers. So is irritability. We remember the W.C. Fields movie in which he reacts rather strongly to the sound of an Alka-Seltzer fizzing in a glass nearby: "Can't anyone do anything about that racket?" he cries out in hungover anguish.

Sleep Is Still the Best Cure: Part of your hangover is caused by the lack of REM (Rapid Eye Movement) sleep, which is the deepest, best and most refreshing part of sleep. It is also the part of sleep which alcohol suppresses. The only cure is to sleep some more.

Vitamins and Minerals: We knew a newspaperman who drank too much as a matter of course. He also took vitamins, especially the B and C vitamins, regularly. He weathered his drinking better than anyone else we ever met. His refrigerator was always crammed full of these vitamins, along with various minerals, especially magnesium, for the morning after. When you drink too much, you consequently urinate too much — and this makes your hangover worse. Our friend took his vitamins both the evening before he began drinking, and the morning after. But he claimed that even if he hadn't taken them the night before, a gulp of B vitamins would do wonders the mornings he woke up with bad hangovers, which were all too many, even he had to admit.

After one of this newspaperman's parties (which he threw often and well) the authors admit they awoke with terrible hangovers. Since the party had been at the newspaperman's house, the authors had spent the night there. The newspaperman took us to the refrigerator door where he stored all his vitamins and minerals, waiting to do combat with the hangover. We tried the cure, and our hangovers lasted a shorter time than others had in the past.

Milk Before Aspirin: While aspirin offers some relief from hangover-induced headaches, it adds to the overall pain. For aspirin is hard on stomachs, and it's especially hard on stomachs that are in agony during hangovers. Better first to force a little milk down your throat, for it will coat and protect your newly-sensitized stomach against fresh assaults by increasing acids.

Dark Rooms: Part of having a bad hangover is the simple fact that you've been oblivious to what your body was trying to tell you the night before when you were up to all your antics, but were too numbed to know what was going on. Living the good life can be exhausting both mentally and physically. If you have pushed yourself too far, rest and recuperation is the prescription you need. You should rest in a darkened room as long as possible — for the whole day if you can.

The Cabbage Cure: Cabbage provides one of the most ancient hangover cures known to man. Wild cabbage was discovered long ago to have the ability to dry out the bad effects of too much drinking. As man invented more and different kinds of liquors, cabbage also became increasingly popular. The Greeks, the English, and the Russians all traditionally included cabbage in their food and drink orgies. The scientific basis to cabbage's fame as a hangover remedy is probably due to the fact that the plant is rich in vitamins and minerals, especially when consumed raw. If you are planning to imbibe, have some fresh cabbage around for the morning. The odds are you're going to need it.

A HOUSEHOLD REMEDY FROM 1865

From a book called *Household Advice,* published in 1865, we have gleaned this wonderful headache cure. "Take a glass jar and half fill the jar with scented rose petals and lavender flowers. Pour white wine vinegar over until the jar is full. Close the jar tightly and place in the sun for about a week. Decant off the liquid and strain through a fine cloth. When needed for a headache place a clean cloth in some of this liquid which has been chilled and apply to your forehead."

DIANNA P.'S NEVER-FAIL HEADACHE CURE

We would like to close this chapter on a very positive note, and tell you about Dianna P.'s headache cure. Dianna believes wholeheartedly in holistic medicine, and she and a friend perfected a cure for headaches that requires two people, but, she says, "It always works for me, and usually works for my friends. In fact, I can't think of anyone it didn't work on."

The person administering the headache remedy starts by giving the sufferer a good neck and upper back massage, not neglecting the muscles under the shoulder blades. After this, the massager should look for the two long tendons in the base of the sufferer's neck; they are about an inch apart, located next to the spine. Right where the spine and the skull meet, at the point where the tendons meet the skull, there are two pressure points. Using his strongest thumb, the massager should press one of those spots for three minutes, applying firm pressure and rotating the tip of the thumb slightly. At the same time, he should press on the front of the sufferer's forehead with his other hand. Repeat the process for the other pressure point; continue for three minutes as before. Now the massager should place his strongest thumb in the hollow between the two long tendons at the base of the skull. The base should be pressed slowly with a slightly rotating motion, while again pressing the front of the forehead with the other hand.

Not so incidentally, we'd like to add that Dianna P. has cured both of us of more than one headache with this remedy.

SUMMARY

There are few of us who have not suffered from headaches. Not only do headaches have many different causes, but many of the causes are in the environment so that there is little we can do about them except to isolate them, and try to avoid them, if possible. Other times headaches can be cured with a nap or a snack. Massage techniques are of great help. And there are also herbal remedies that can banish those headaches.

6

THE POWERFUL
HEALING BENEFITS
OF HOT AND COLD WATER

Generally speaking, the authors of this book are the kind of people who are suspicious of overly simplified or too obvious solutions to health problems. So, when we heard that water — the plain, simple, ubiquitous liquid made up of two parts hydrogen and one part oxygen — could cure what ails you, we were frankly skeptical. Then one of the authors experienced a vivid demonstration of how water therapy can, indeed, perform miracles, and became an amazed convert to hydrotherapy.

What happened was this: One winter a large portion of the population of Los Angeles was laid low by flu. It seemed that no one was able to avoid it. Neither of the authors of this book proved an exception to this rule, unfortunately. One of the side effects of this flu was constipation. It came on towards the end of the illness, as the flu was running its course. In the case of one of the authors, the constipation precipitated another, far more serious, problem; agonizing pain whenever he tried to have a bowel movement.

This unbelievable pain drove the sufferer to a local doctor. What the doctor's examination revealed was not that the author had a case of hemorrhoids, but a severe anal ulcer, a yawning fissure in the rectum. A second consultation, with a high-priced Beverly Hills proctologist, ended up rather predictably — the specialist strongly recommended an operation. But writers don't make enough money to be able to afford expensive surgical procedures, so the author regretfully had to decline. He next took himself over to the UCLA Medical Clinic in Westwood to be examined. They told him that an operation might not be a bad idea, but that recovering from it would most likely be as bad as the pain stemming from the original problem. While recovering from the operation, the author would have to live in his bathtub; whereas, if he did nothing about getting the operation in the first place, the fissure would likely heal itself.

It was definitely a case of "Hobson's choice." Unable (and unwilling) to undergo the operation, the author sequestered himself in his bathtub at home, for he soon found that every time he got out of the tub, the pain became unbearable, even with various prescription painkillers. Gradually, he began to notice that the pain was subsiding, bit by bit, until finally he was able to spend more and more time out of the tub. By the end of two weeks, the pain was completely gone. Not only had the hot water of the bathtub kept the severe pain of the anal ulcer at a manageable level, but it had obviously speeded up the healing process as well. If it hadn't been for hot water, the author doubts very much whether he would have survived those hellish weeks.

THE ANCIENT IMPORTANCE OF WATER

The ancients were aware of how important water was. Although in ancient Egypt only the very rich could afford baths, in ancient India there were great public baths. The enormous public baths excavated at the archeological digs in Mohenjo-Daro and Harappa, India, showed that plumbing technology was quite sophisticated as much as 5,000 years ago. The Mohenjo-Daro public bath had a drain and underground pipes, so that the water could be changed. There were also steam baths, fountains, and other bathing accoutrements. What was most interesting about this archeological discovery was that it dated back before the invasion of India by the Aryan Hindus, and also long before the time of the Greeks and Romans, who were believed to be the arch-bathers of ancient times.

Natural hot springs have always been favorite places for both humans and animals to soak their weary bones. The early Romans took bathing one step further and built massive stone baths in the form of huge mosaic temples, which were socializing centers for Roman society.

The Greeks took short, cold baths as part of their athletic regime. The Turks, on the other hand, appreciated the luxuries of heat and steam. The Finns and Swedes, of course, specialized in dry-heat saunas. The religious ceremonies of Moslems, Hindus, and Jews required ritual bathing — water has had religious significance from the dawn of civilization.

King Henry IV of England founded the Order of the Bath to teach his knights to bathe regularly; the knights

111

were encouraged in their personal cleanliness by pretty wenches who aided them in the bath, and the water was perfumed by the addition of rose petals. Later on, however, things took a turn for the worse when Christian zealots (including members of the Church of England and the American Puritans) went largely unwashed because baths were associated with licentiousness and nudity.

The Japanese have always made a fetish of very hot baths, typically emerging from them "red as a boiled octopus." In Europe, doctors have long recommended bathing for health and pleasure. The most famous European spas are in Bath, England; Baden-Baden, West Germany; and Aix-les-Bains in the French Alps. There are similar spas in the United States, such as Saratoga Springs in New York State and many hot springs in Southern California. As a youngster, one of the authors used to luxuriate on weekends at Seminole Hot Springs, in the Malibu mountains just north of Los Angeles, where sulphur was the chief ingredient in the water.

In the nineteenth century, author Robert Louis Stevenson, who suffered all his life from poor health, went to Calistoga Springs, California, on his honeymoon. He attributed his improved health to the hot springs and warm climate.

THE "MAGIC" OF HOT WATER

Many early cultures commonly believed that there was something "magical" about spring waters — many of the skeletons recovered from ancient geothermal areas show a high number of fractures and breaks in their bones. Apparently the wounded were hoping that the "magic" water would heal them.

In the early part of this century, there were literally hundreds of natural spring resorts where hot baths, massages, and other water treatments were common.

But it is entirely possible that the curative effects of hot springs can be obtained as easily in your bathtub at home as it can be at an expensive or far-flung mineral spa. The "magic" of a hot springs, the experts suspect, lies in the fact that the heat of the water raises body temperature. Just as your body temperature increases when you get sick, and the healing process is accelerated, so does the temperature rise when you immerse yourself in hot water — and the healing process can take place more rapidly. If your home hot water heater is working well, you can accomplish the same thing in your bathtub as you can at a health spa — just turn on the water faucet as hot as you can stand it.

WHY MILLIONS OF GERMANS TAKE THE "CURE"

West Germany has a system of some 252 spas, which are inspected and regulated by the government. Germans are taking to the water in an even bigger way than they did in the past. They are going to the baths because they have discovered that the waters revitalize their tired and aching bodies, and "sweep away the mental cobwebs and stress of daily life." Every two years, German citizens are given a three or four week cure at public expense at one of the spas — and the time isn't even counted against regular vacation time! The Germans obviously feel they are on to something, and you might be well advised to consider the same for yourself. Our country has not yet fully taken to the healing powers of water in so dramatic a way, although hot tubs, jacuzzis and even swimming pools perhaps attest to the fact that we are taking to the water too, just in our own particular style.

In Germany, labor unions and employers alike believe in the preventive cures afforded by hot water. Eugen Wannenwetsch of the Munich University medical facility believes that for every dollar spent sending a worker to a hot water cure, three dollars are saved in making the worker more efficient on his job and less likely to take off time for sick leave.

The German water cure spas are all located near mineral or hot springs, some of which have been in use since Roman times. One such bath, Bad Neuenahr, with its iron-rich springs reaching temperatures up to 100 degrees Fahrenheit, is used in the treatment of diabetes and other metabolic disorders, diseases of the liver and urinary tract, and diseases of the heart and circulatory system. The baths are also good for all kinds of nervous exhaustion, neuralgic pains, and muscular ailments.

Most of our readers are not likely to jump on the next flight to Bad Neuenahr to be pummeled by a masseur, blasted with high-pressure water hoses, or encouraged to sweat it out in the spa's sauna, so we will tell you how some German techniques utilizing water can be used in your own bathtub. Water, although it may be growing scarcer and more expensive, is still far cheaper than international air travel.

USING YOUR TUB TO REDUCE FEVER

If you're running a rather high fever, take a cold bath and stay in the tub for as long as you can. This method was originally discovered more than a century ago during an epidemic of typhus. The patients were given a cold bath while also receiving a constant massage. Many patients survived who would have otherwise died from the disease. One authority was quoted at the time as saying, "Cold bathing is a power for good, before which all other measures must stand outside."

The cold water treatment should be reserved only for those with high temperatures. When you are getting out of the tub, make sure you have big comfortable towels to thoroughly dry yourself off and a warm, toasty bed to get into. The reader should exercise caution with this method, and do so only in consultation with his or her doctor.

FIGHTING COLDS WITH WATER

There are things you can do with water to fight colds. To begin with, you can drink the stuff. But another way you can avoid catching colds when you first feel the symptoms coming on is to exercise, and then step into a hot tub. At the same time apply a cold compress to the forehead. By tradition, hot baths have been shown to be effective for sufferers of arthritis, bronchitis, gall bladder problems, gout, and muscle aches as well as colds.

IMPROVING PERISTALSIS WITH WATER

If you are one of those people plagued with a sluggish peristaltic action, start the day by drinking cold water. Do so first thing in the morning and continue throughout the day. If you're sitting in a restaurant, drink that glass of cold ice water. You also will get a good jolt to get your system going the first thing in the morning, not only by drinking cold water, but also by plunging your feet into cold water as well. We've done it with a pan by the side of the bed.

People frequently forget to drink enough water. The result is sometimes constipation. You can probably avoid that constipation simply by drinking more water throughout the day. That glass of cold water is a treat you should learn not to refuse. Say you've been out walking, and it is a hot day. Your muscles feel weak. What is happening is that you are suffering from a slight case of dehydration. A glass or two of water will fix you up. Remember, most of the time drinking lots of water cannot be harmful to you — unless you really go overboard and drink until you burst, which isn't likely.

HOW TO SOOTHE AND SOFTEN ITCHY SKIN

Bran and your bathtub can cure various skin problems and relieve itchy skin. Take several handfuls of bran and sew them into a cheesecloth pouch. Soak the pouch with its contents in hot water in your tub for several minutes, then fill the rest of the bathtub with regular warm bath water. The bath water will turn a milky color. Relax in the tub for as long as you can.

Adding sodium bicarbonate and ordinary laundry starch to bath water will also help with various skin problems.

A NEW USE FOR VITAMIN C

Vitamin C has been credited with curing all kinds of ailments, but possibly one of the most surprising is the suggestion of pouring ascorbic acid into the bathtub as a treatment for hemorrhoids. Incidentally, a lot of people are under the misapprehension that only secretaries and others such as writers, who lead what is generally called a sedentary life, suffer from this malady, but sad to report for the rest of you out there, this isn't so. Physically

116

active people, such as athletes and dancers, are also predisposed towards hemorrhoids. It was an athletic consultant for the Denver Broncos and Denver Nuggets, Dr. John Hanks, who claims to have greatly speeded up the hemorrhoid healing process by adding ascorbic acid to the athletes' baths. Hanks advocates adding a cup of ascorbic acid powder for every five quarts of cool water, and then staying in the bath for up to fifteen minutes at a time.

All the proctologists spoken to by the author of this book who suffered from the anal fissure were unanimous in saying that one particular brand of hemorrhoid relief medication — the most famous of them all — was neither effective nor safe, despite advertising to the contrary.

CURING INCONTINENCE
WITH YOUR GARDEN HOSE

Various methods of directing a shower of water toward one specific part of the body have been found to be of great value in curing a number of different ailments. For example, applying a stream of water from your garden hose, perhaps with the addition of a shower head or other nozzle, directly to the soles of the feet, can reduce the embarrassment of incontinence in older people. A jet stream of water should be directed at the soles of the feet for up to two minutes. This also helps reduce the suffering that comes from having cold feet, as the spray of water increases circulation in the area.

AN UNUSUAL HEMORRHOID CURE

Geri M. cured her bleeding hemorrhoids with witch hazel and warm water. Her doctor had suggested that she have an operation, but she had to support her three sons and couldn't afford the time or expense involved in such an undertaking. So her doctor suggested an alternative remedy — to add a quarter of a cup of witch hazel to a basin full of warm water, and sit in it as long as possible whenever possible. Within three days Geri's problems were gone. The bleeding had stopped and all her symptoms had disappeared. That, she said, was forty years ago — and she has not had a recurrence since then.

MORE JET STREAM REMEDIES

Ying S. had problems with constipation. She was afraid of becoming hooked on laxatives, so when she heard of the following technique, she tried it. It was nothing more complex than directing a steam of cold water to the abdominal area. Ying would get up first thing in the morning, don her bathing suit, and march out to the back yard. Everyone in the house had left already; Ying had a job that didn't start until later — banker's hours, she used to joke. Yet she was also an early riser, and a non-stop tinkerer. What she had rigged up, from her husband's carpentry shop, was a simple wooden frame that held the hose pointed at her abdomen. She used this for about a week and her constipation simply disapeared. She felt it coming back again about two weeks later, so she gave herself the treatment again. She hasn't had much occasion to use the hose technique in quite a while since then. The wooden device still stands in her back yard, for whenever Ying begins to feel a case of constipation coming on, she puts the garden hose back in its little holder and lets it work its strange cure.

The device described above is *homemade*. It is, of course, therefore not available commercially. Something similar could be built by the reader for use in his bathroom if he wanted to bring the hose in through the bathroom window.

Ying also discovered that various aches and pains in her bladder, uterus and pelvic areas also responded favorably to the abdominal shower method. Alternating hot and cold streams of water also will help lower back problems, as well as chronic diarrhea and other digestive upsets.

BARBARA'S HEADACHE CURE

Barbara was plagued with headaches. She found that she could keep them at bay, however, by spraying cold water on her entire feet in an on-and-off again fashion. She told us that after doing this two or three times a day, ten or fifteen minutes each time, for six months, there has been no reappearance of her former headaches.

SOME ASSORTED OTHER WATER REMEDIES

The Digestion Cure: If you have a sudden attack of indigestion, try drinking a large amount of warm water for fast relief. Warm water cleanses the stomach and dilutes the excess hydrochloric acid that is likely to be causing the problem. Hot compresses applied externally on the area where the pain is concentrated will also help; apply a fresh compress every ten minutes. Remember, however, that acute indigestion can signal appendicitis, so if you're ever in doubt, do not attempt home treatment — see your doctor at once.

A Great Way to Sweat Out Insomnia: If you suffer from insomnia, warm tubs can help relax you into a good night's sleep. Applying a hot, moist compress to the head should make you even drowsier. Some of the most wonderfully complete sleeps the authors have ever been privileged to enjoy came when we spent part of a summer in a cabin in rural, wooded Topanga Canyon, which is only a few miles away from busy Hollywood. Our sound sleep may have been attributable to the fact that we were waking up to the sounds of birds rustling in trees, clear blue skies, and no traffic or other unpleasant urban noises. But another major factor had to be the wonderful hot tub in which we soaked before going to sleep every night. Beneath the starry night sky, we'd soak there in the tub, which was a wooden one made from the noble redwood.

Compresses: Compresses are nothing more than pieces of cloth soaked in either hot or cold water, then wrung out and applied somewhere on the body. Hot compresses relieve pain, soreness, and swellings. Cold ones help reduce fevers and aid in reducing the pain of hemorrhoids.

Cold compresses constrict the capillary blood vessels, which connect with the major arteries, and are thus useful in reducing fever. They should be placed under the arms and on the forehead. Hot compresses, on the other hand, relax muscles and are effective pain killers. Immerse the towel in hot water; wring out the extra water, and place on the affected area. Change every five minutes or so for at least 30 minutes.

EUROPEAN WATER CURES
FOR ARTHRITIS

It's a little far from home, but next time you're traveling around the world and you want to do something about your arthritis, make a stop in Yugoslavia, Greece,

Rumania, or Israel, where arthritis is treated with hot water. In these countries, it is traditional for the arthritis sufferer to take a hot bath just before bedtime. There are also spas where people go to soak in the water for days because the water improves painful conditions. So if you want to get out of your own home for a while, there's a spa in the Dead Sea that's been used by arthritis sufferers since the time of Julius Caesar. On the other hand, if you can't afford to travel, stick with the hot baths at night.

A DOCTOR'S WATER THERAPY SUGGESTIONS FOR RENEWED HEALTH AND VIGOR

One of the foremost practitioners of water therapy in Southern California was Victor H. Lindlahr, who operated a sanitarium in the area some years ago. Lindlahr's son Henry, a medical doctor, wrote about his father's various water treatments in a book called *The Natural Way to Health.* A selection of a few of his treatments follow.

Circulation Problems: Lindlahr recommends a vapor bath. The bathroom is to be warmly heated, but the tub filled with cold water. In Lindlahr's sanitarium, there were professional attendants. But your spouse will do if you are doing this in your own house. The person steps into the tub and fills his cupped hands full of water, which is then splashed on the right leg, and the leg rubbed. This process is repeated on the left leg, the chest, and both arms, taking no longer than one minute in each area. It is obviously important to dry yourself thoroughly right afterwards so as not to catch pneumonia.

Throbbing Headaches: The good doctor's recommendation for these was a cold sitz bath, with eight inches of water. You squat in it until your hips are under the water. Count to ten, get out, dry off, and lie down for a few minutes. This should get rid of headache pain within minutes. On the other hand, if your headache is a dull, continuous pain located mainly at the back of the head, take a hot sitz bath, using eight inches of water. Recline in the hot water for ten or fifteen minutes, then get out, dry yourself, and lie down. "The pain will have been relieved as if by magic," Dr. Lindlahr promised.

Blood pressure: A hot bath was prescribed; this would reduce the blood pressure by as much as 15 percent, said Lindlahr.

For the Curse of Migraines: Squatting in eight inches of hot water for twenty minutes or so was recommended.

Varicose Veins: Standing in cold water up to the calves for a couple of minutes was suggested. Then dry yourself with a coarse towel, and walk about briskly.

Hair Growth: Hair could be encouraged to grow, said Dr. Lindlahr, by running lots of cold water on it, then vigorously pinching and massaging the scalp with your fingertips while the water is running. He added, however, that you should dry yourself thoroughly afterward to avoid catching cold.

Prostate Problem Cramps: Men who have prostate problems also sometimes suffer from cramps. For these, Dr. Lindlahr said lukewarm sitz baths were best.

Hot Flashes: Women who suffer from this problem should step into a bath with two inches of cold water in it. They should splash around vigorously for several minuts without actually sitting down. Then the feet should be dried and rubbed, and the woman should walk briskly around the room.

7

HEALING HANDS: DIGITAL RELIEF FOR WHAT AILS YOU

In the earlier chapters of this book, you learned how common ailments could be cured by simple, easy-to-use home remedies incorporating ingredients you already had around the house. Now we are going to look at some remedies for common ailments which don't require anything more than your fingertips.

You are probably familiar with the amazing science of acupuncture, but did you know that you can treat yourself at home using the basic principles of acupuncture without acupuncture needles?

For thousands of years, mankind has been aware of the seemingly unrelated but actually inextricably interwoven relationships between various pressure points on the outside of the body and the internal organs. Perhaps the fledgling science of acupressure began one day long ago when someone undergoing an anxiety attack realized that biting hard on his lower lip suddenly reduced the nervousness to a more manageable level. As long as a thousand years ago the ancient Chinese were fully aware of hundreds of pressure points on the body and had systematic charts showing which area controlled which bodily functions and ailments.

Nowadays there are a number of needleless acupressure systems that enable the patient to safely self-treat many ailments using only the fingers. These systems are perfectly safe; all that is required is an understanding of the main pressure points and the organs or functions which these control.

TONI W.'S STRESS, TENSION, INSOMNIA, AND NIGHTMARE CURE

Toni W., a young woman in her mid-twenties, had a great deal of stress in her life and as a result found herself lying awake into the wee small hours trying to fall asleep. When she finally did drop off, she usually suffered from such horrible nightmares that she almost always started wide awake, and the vicious circle would begin all over again.

She confided her problem to her mother, who knew a great deal about acupressure techniques, and her mother immediately applied an acupressure massage technique which not only worked immediately but also kept Toni relaxed for a number of days afterward.

The massage was applied to both the procephalic pulses, which you can locate for yourself by feeling along your temples until you find the rounded curves of your forehead. Gentle pressure was applied to both of these points using one finger from each hand for each point. Because Toni was under so much stress, her mother suggested that she also drop her jaw during the massage, which lasted for about a minute. After thirty seconds,

Toni experienced a pleasurable tingling on the top of her head, and total relaxation swiftly followed. Now whenever she experiences a return of the stressful situation that originally caused her insomnia and resulting tension, she self-administers this healing massage. She has not been troubled by the problem since.

HOW TO PUT THIS SIMPLE SYSTEM
TO WORK FOR YOU

Though there are a number of different types of pressure point therapies, their proponents all agree on one basic fact: they work. Some authorities recommend gentle pressure, others more vigorous pressure, but in treating simple ailments it is wise not to overdo it. Begin massaging gently at first; only increase the pressure if you feel you are not getting results.

To begin applying this simple form of self-healing, locate the appropriate point. These will be described a little later. Remember that these pressure points are rarely very large, and that if you happen to overshoot a bit you will not be applying pressure to the correct area for your problem.

You will probably notice right away if you have hit on the right pressure point. It may feel bruised or tender or it may offer some resistance. Even so, it is not a good idea to press down very hard; exercise restraint, especially if you are just beginning to use this method of treatment.

You should place the tip of your index finger or your thumb on the point or points, pressing down firmly but gently. If two points require stimulation, use the same finger on each hand for each of them. While you are pressing down, vibrate your finger(s) slightly in order to apply a light massage to the area.

Some authorities recommend the use of such auxiliary massage devices as the end of a ballpoint pen or a thimble; and as long as you are gentle there is really no harm in employing them. But the most sensitive massager remains your own finger. Only you can judge which method is the best one for you.

RELIEF FROM COMMON AILMENTS
IS AT YOUR FINGERTIPS

Next time you find yourself suffering from a bout of indigestion or excess stomach acid, don't automatically reach for that drugstore remedy. Instead, massage the center of the sole of one foot for nine or ten minutes, using your fingertips. Relief should be immediate.

Likewise, constipation, even long-standing and obstinate constipation, with or without the annoying and embarrassing flatulence that so often accompanies it, will respond wonderfully to acupressure techniques. Apply the massage to the area in the center of the chin just below the lower lip; if you feel around with your fingers you will easily be able to locate it. Keep it up for a few minutes; you will most likely experience a complete evacuation of the bowels in fifteen minutes.

There are a number of ways to get rid of headaches using acupressure massage. For a headache that strikes sudenly, press on your forehead about half an inch above the bridge of your nose for nine or ten minutes. Another method of curing a headache is to stick out your tongue half an inch or so and bite down hard on it for nine minutes. It is not advisable to continue biting your tongue in this manner for more than eleven minutes.

A stiff neck can make your whole day wretched. To solve this knotty problem, massage the bottom of your foot (either foot) just above the base of your little toe. Repeat the massage three times daily to ensure that the problem does not continue.

The bottom of the foot is also the acupressure massage site for curing hiccups. When an attack comes on, rub the sole of the foot fairly vigorously for nine or ten minutes, focusing on the center of the sole.

MORE ACUPRESSURE POINT REMEDIES
FOR COMMON COMPLAINTS

The following remedies do not necessarily employ fingertip acupressure massage, but they are based on the same acupressure points nonetheless.

For headaches, try pressing your thumb firmly against the roof of your mouth; hold it there for three to five minutes. If the ache covers an extensive portion of your head, you may need to shift the position of your thumb around until you have covered the entire area.

If you tend to suffer from bouts of motion sickness or "sick stomach," carry a wire hairbrush and a metal comb with you wherever you travel. At the first suggestion of queasiness, begin applying pressure to the backs of the hands with the teeth of the metal comb. Run the comb across the area extending from the thumb and first finger, including the web of skin between the thumb and first finger. Relief will be forthcoming in five to ten minutes.

After eating a heavy meal, are you troubled by a feeling of sluggishness, centering around your stomach? Try gently stroking your wire hairbrush across the backs of your hands for a few minutes. Both this and the previous remedy can be applied using the fingernails, but quicker relief has been observed to result from the use of metal.

HOW RUTH U. ELIMINATED
MIGRAINE HEADACHES

Ruth U. had suffered from migraine headaches since she was an early teenager. The condition came on without any warning and caused her indescribable pain for three or four days without letup. Needless to say, she dreaded the arrival of these migraine attacks and tried many different remedies to combat them, none of which worked.

Finally she consulted a naturopathic doctor, who took one look at her and immediately used acupressure therapy. He applied massage to her forehead for nine minutes twice a week for three months. At the end of the first three months, Ruth was experiencing no pain whatsoever; after five years, she was still migraine-free.

SOME "POINTS" TO REMEMBER

Bear in mind that acupressure massage therapy, while amazingly potent, cannot treat health problems arising from secondary causes. For instance, if you find that acupressure massage technique is not curing an obstinate case of constipation, the chances are good that your constipation is the result of poor diet, insufficient exercise, or flabby abdominal muscles. Remember that the best way to remain healthy is to eat a balanced diet, get plenty of daily exercise, and resist temptations and excesses such as overconsumption of alcohol, tobacco, or drugs. If you have a health problem that does not immediately respond to acupressure massage correctly applied, discontinue the massage at once and consult a physician.

SUMMARY

Acupressure massage techniques cover a broad spectrum of health problems. To employ them accurately for almost any common ailment, you need to know the complete acupressure point system. There are many books which list the entire system in more detail than we can here. Check at your local health food store or library.

8

THE GENTLE ART
OF RELAXING MOVEMENT

Strenuous and demanding exercise typified by jogging has nothing to do with the relaxing movement mentioned in the title of this chapter. The movement we are referring to is gentle, subtle, very civilized and Oriental in conception.

Thousands of years of Eastern philosophy ultimately led to an ethic of balance and moderation. Although the twentieth century has, regrettably perhaps, seen a major trend toward Westernization sweeping countries such as Japan, with a corresponding fascination with American sports, nonetheless the Eastern philosophy remains remarkably serene. That serenity extends itself to exercise and even, oddly enough, to the practice of Oriental martial arts. Paradoxical as it might seem to a Westerner who has been raised with images of aggression and resistance when it comes to self-defense, Oriental martial arts focus not on aggression but on stability, balance and a sense of centeredness, enabling the initiate to defend himself by remaining continuously aware of his opponent's strengths and weaknesses.

While you may not be able or willing to rush out to enroll in a Tai Chi Chu'an class or start studying karate or judo, you can formulate a simple, comfortable personalized exercise program that utilizes the spirit of moderation inherent in Eastern philosophy. Exercise need not be unpleasant, exhausting and miserable; by taking a leaf out of the book of Eastern wisdom you can enjoy the benefits of regular exercise without falling prey to its excesses.

HOW SIMPLE MOVEMENTS WILL INCREASE YOUR WELL-BEING

As has already been suggested above, to begin your personalized movement program, the first thing you need to do is change your conception of what exercise really is. Once you have banished the specter of exercise as a sweaty, unpleasant enterprise, you will be well on the road to positive change.

To accomplish this change, consider for a moment some of the benefits of regular exercise. Many scientific studies have shown that regular exercise greatly improves the well-being of the exerciser; those who exercise regularly tend to show less depression, lower blood pressure, better-regulated appetites, and less insomnia, and have numerous other signs of glowing good health.

The case of Maurice L. graphically illustrates what regular mild exercise can do for a person. Our friend Maurice was a rather corpulent fellow in his mid-thirties who found himself feeling sluggish and somewhat depressed. Because he earned his living as a bartender, he consequently spent a great deal of time standing up but not actually moving around. His sluggishness sent him to his doctor, who, after ruling out any physical ailment, recommended regular exercise. At first Maurice was skeptical; he was hardly the outdoors type, and he had never had much enthusiasm for sports. What could he do that would qualify as exercise? A suggestion from his doctor finally solved the problem: how about a daily walk around Maurice's neighborhood? Maurice agreed to try this, so for the next week he forced himself to stroll about a mile every day. By the end of the week he was amazed to find that he had a great deal of energy he'd never known he possessed. It was no trouble to continue his walking for another week; by the end of the second week, he reported to his doctor that he had dropped five pounds without missing a single meal! After he had been getting regular exercise for a month, Maurice's depression had all but evaporated. Even the sad stories of some of his customers were unable to bring it back.

A SIMPLE PATH TO HEALTH
AND LONG LIFE

As we have seen in the case of Maurice L., the best solution was the simplest solution. Part of Maurice's problem was the nature of his work: regular exercise, however, introduced him to a more balanced way of life, and that, in turn, enabled him to offset the physical and mental difficulties he faced as a result of his job.

You probably don't need a doctor to tell you what you already know — the key to good health is regularity in your habits and the avoidance of habitual overindulgences such as too much alcohol, greasy or spicy foods, or refined starches and sugars. But too stringent an approach is equally inadvisable. To stay healthy, you need to be able to stick with your routine. For that reason, the exercise suggestions that follow will not be especially overtaxing; we want you to continue practicing them. The best exercise program in the world won't help a bit if you don't keep it up. The idea underlying this philosophy is to feel comfortable with what you are doing. If you feel the least bit uncomfortable, you'll probably give up.

GETTING STARTED BY RELAXING

Prepare yourself to begin to exercise by breathing deeply. Deep breathing, if correctly practiced, will relax your entire body and free it from stress and tension. Close your eyes and lie on a bed or on a thick rug with your head on a high pillow. Breathe slowly and deeply, inhaling and exhaling about six times per minute. Be sure to relax your chest by allowing your diaphragm and stomach muscles to do most of the work. Exhale through your mouth, not through your nose; press lightly on your abdomen to release the air. Continue for five or ten minutes, or until you begin to feel relaxed.

RELAXING YOUR BODY FROM
HEAD TO TOE

Now you can stand up and slowly start to exercise. Since this is a gradual movement program, we aren't going to suggest that you suddenly sprint out the door and gallop down the street. Instead, we will lead you through a progressive series of movements that will get your circulation going and your heart beating steadily.

The first of these movements is intended to relax the trunk. This part of the body often reflects pent-up tension by the presence of backache, difficulties with breathing, or even chest pains. Once you have relaxed your trunk and banished any tension that may have built up there, you will be able to continue your progressive movement program.

To relax the trunk, stand in a loose, comfortable position, neither excessively rigid nor excessively lax. Your back should be straight but not stiff and your feet should be slightly apart. Rub your hands together to warm them, and gently massage the lower abdominal region with either hand, using a circular motion. Massage this area thirty-six times, then repeat the massage another thirty-six times, using the left hand.

Now, remaining in the same relaxed posture, rub your lower back with the backs of both hands simultaneously. Do this fifty times. Begin the lower back massage slightly above the lower back area, slanting the hands toward one another and meeting in the middle of the lower back.

Now that your trunk is relaxed, you can engage in a little relaxed standing. Move your feet apart until the distance of their separation is equal to the width of your shoulders. They should be directly opposite one another, and the toes should point forward. Your head, neck and trunk should be in a straight line, with the central point being the soles of your feet. Be sure to remain relaxed but not too loose. Let your hands drop down next to your thighs with their backs forward.

Now breathe deeply and look straight ahead. Remain standing in this manner for five or ten minutes, always breathing deeply and evenly. If you feel tension in any part of your body, or if you experience a cramp or any other discomfort, temporarily abandon the posture and massage the affected area before you resume standing again.

WALKING CAN DO WONDERS

Now you should be sufficiently relaxed to do a little walking. At first remember not to over-exert yourself. Try a leisurely walk around the block for the first couple of times, then gradually increase the amount of walking to three or four blocks. What is important is the fact that you should be getting regular daily exercise; at this point the amount of exercise you get is not as important as the fact that you are getting it regularly.

While walking, balance the weight of your body on one foot at a time, and alternate feet smoothly. Keep your strides brisk but not rushed; bear in mind the old Chinese adage that effective walking resembles that of a pigeon strutting along in a sprightly fashion. Keep the body straight, but not rigid, and the mind empty of tense or unpleasant thoughts. Breathe deeply and smoothly.

During the hot summer months you can replace or augment your walking with a daily swim, if you own a swimming pool or have access to a public pool. Swimming is by far the best single exercise known to man. A single half hour of wholehearted swimming can not only cool you off and relax you, it can also burn off as many calories as would be burned by jogging, without any of the injurious side effects of the latter. Just remember not to overdo it; you should be looking forward to repeating the exercise again the next day, not looking for excuses to get out of it.

MICHAEL D.'S EASY PROGRAM
FOR A ROBUST CONSTITUTION

Michael D., an anemic, underweight young man, was so run-down that he had no energy for much of anything. Despite receiving treatment for his anemia (which was partly due to an ill-thought-out vegetarian diet, later remedied), Michael realized that he needed exercise. He was a voracious reader of self-help and health books and magazines, and since at that time many of these were advocating jogging, he decided to go along with it. However, despite expensive running shoes, this only landed him in a podiatrist's office with aches and pains in his feet and ankles.

With his visions of someday being a marathon runner so cruelly deflated, Michael turned back to books and magazines for inspiration. Since he was unable to run, and his jogging injuries made walking unfeasible, at least until they healed, he investigated the benefits of yoga. He looked up a few simple beginners' yoga positions, and after a couple weeks' practice he began to breathe more deeply as a matter of course as well as sleeping better at night. After a month he began to experience energy reserves he never suspected he had. Gradually he added more exercises, and eventually his daily program lasted about forty-five minutes. Today, Michael is a yoga instructor in Hollywood; the old, run-down Michael of bygone days is no longer.

Michael recommends the following simple yoga exercises for beginners who are interested in slowly building a personal exercise plan. Yoga is a vast and complex system, and if you are serious about studying it beyond these few beginning exercises, you should find yourself a qualified teacher. But by adding these exercises to your daily program you cannot harm yourself, and, on the contrary, you will become more supple and graceful.

The first exercise is a simple one, known as "The Mountain." Like the earlier exercises mentioned above, this is not an especially strenuous exercise. Stand in front of a full-length mirror; stand up straight, with your weight distributed evenly between both feet. Be sure your knees are firm and in a straight line with your calves. Your spine should be held erectly, with your head balanced over it. Relax your shoulders and abdominal area. Hold this pose for a few minutes, observing yourself in the mirror while you do so.

You may be saying, "So much for the rigors of yoga practice!" but consider this: The "Mountain" pose is far more subtle than you probably realize. This seemingly simple posture actually reveals more about you than you might imagine. For example, if you find that you tend to stand with your weight thrown back on your heels, this indicates that you are easily knocked off-balance; any sudden disturbance could cause both your mind and body to lose their center of gravity, with the consequent result that you might also lose control of your life. If you noticed that you have a tendency to thrust your head or your entire body forward, you may approach life from a too aggressive standpoint; or perhaps you have an inferiority complex and are attempting to remedy it by adopting an over-compensatory pose. Either way, you should relax and attempt to overcome this rigid attitude.

If you stood with your chest in a caved-in position, you might have problems expressing yourself fluently, or you may lack self-confidence and be unable to approach others without feeling somehow inferior. Conversely, if you found that you threw out your chest, you may have an egotistical view of yourself or of your abilities — or perhaps wish you did.

The "Mountain" pose is extremely valuable in allowing you to diagnose your state of mind as it relates to the state of your body. And that, of course, is yoga's greatest strength — it enables you to forge a strong link between your body and your mind, and understand just how the two interact.

Our next basic yoga position is a little more active than the previous one. Called the "Triangle," it strengthens your thigh and lower leg muscles and loosens up the torso. Stand with your feet spread widely apart and planted firmly on the floor. Your head should be held erect. Begin by taking a deep breath and then exhaling. Now bend from the waist, being careful to keep your back straight but not stiff. Place your right hand on your left ankle, and raise your left arm up in a straight line, pointing your fingers toward the ceiling. If you feel any stiffness in your neck, move out of the pose and then move back into it again. Most important, you should not feel any muscular discomfort in this position. If you do, it may indicate that you shouldn't be attempting it. However, if done correctly, the "Triangle" pose will not harm your muscles in any way and will in fact lead to improved muscle tone. Remain in the pose for a few minutes, as long as you feel comfortable.

Finally, Michael D. recommends that you try the "Corpse" pose. This is a deceptively easy one, since all that is required is that you lie flat on your back with your hands facing upward, lightly clenched. When you try it, however, you will discover that it is not as easy as you thought it was. The purpose behind this position is to get you to quiet down internally — something which many people find almost impossible to do in these crazy days of tension and overloaded schedules. You must remain in this position for ten to fifteen minutes, during which time you should not attempt to concentrate on anything, but rather to clear your mind of chaos, jangled nerves, depression — anything that happens to be there. Once you have practiced this pose a few times, you will discover that it will greatly benefit your mind and body, whether you are actually doing it at the moment or not. It puts you directly in touch with the serenity that lies at the core of everyone's mind, and that serenity will relax the body as well as the psyche.

For those of you have gone through the simple yoga exercise program above and feel confident that you have mastered the exercises, here are some further, more advanced exercises to try. Do not attempt the following exercises until you feel comfortable with the previous ones; remember that the keyword in this sort of exercise is moderation; do not push yourself or force yourself to accomplish things before you are ready for them.

Neck Stretcher: This exercise is good for warming up the neck and the top of the spinal column before you get into some of the more demanding exercises which will follow.

Stand up straight; with your arms outstretched and your palms facing upward. Lower your right ear onto your right shoulder. Now tilt your head all the way back, then lower your left ear onto your left shoulder. Finally, allow your face to fall all the way forward in front.

When you have gone through these motions a few times, try to pass through the whole sequence of motions continuously and smoothly, rolling your head in a 360-degree circle. Roll clockwise, then counter-clockwise. Repeat the neck stretcher in both directions three or four times.

Deep Breathing: Along with the Neck Stretcher, this exercise will help you warm up and activate your entire nervous system. Stand up straight, with your arms at your sides. Exhale through your nose. Now raise your arms slightly and begin inhaling slowly while at the same time you begin rising off the floor onto your toes. Meanwhile, while rising off the floor, ball your hands into loose fists; raise them tightly into your chest just below your ribcage. Remain in this position about ten seconds with your lungs full of air; then begin slowly to exhale, at the same time lowering your heels back onto the floor and allowing your arms to fall slowly back to your sides. This exercise should be repeated three or four times during your daily exercise routine as well as at the beginning of each exercise session.

Falling Forward: Once again, stand up straight. Bend forward from the waist and, allowing your body to be pulled forward by gravity, let the upper part of your body and your arms fall forward until your fingertips are almost touching the floor. Stay in this position for about five seconds with your chin tucked in toward your throat. Now straighten up, resuming the initial posture. Repeat this exercise three or four times.

Chorus Girl Exercise: Stand up straight with both hands on your hips. Lift your left leg up straight in front

145

of you. Hold it there for a few seconds, then, with your foot sole up in front of you, swing your leg around until it is extended straight out at your left side; hold it in that position for a few seconds. Finally, swing the leg around behind you, still holding it straight out. Hold for a few seconds, then lower it to the ground. Repeat the sequence of motions with your right leg. Exercise each leg twice.

SUMMARY

Exercise need not be a hateful chore that you find yourself putting off every day. This chapter has shown you how to approach exercise mentally in order to build your own personalized exercise formula.

Remember that the important thing about exercise is to engage in it regularly. Doctors recommend that you have three fifteen-to-twenty-minute periods of exercise every week; some of that should ideally be active, such as swimming or brisk walking. Ultimately, however, you are the only judge of what sort of exercise you can keep up with, and what sort of exercise makes you feel the best. The best exercise program in the world will not do you one bit of good if you don't continue with it.

The mind and the body are virtually inseparable in the effects they have on each other, and Eastern wisdom shows that what is good for one is good for the other, and vice versa. Remember in structuring your exercise program that anything that makes you feel bad physically is likely to affect your mental state as well. Thus, you may find that regular exercise will eventually banish depression and fatigue and give you a much more positive outlook on life. Try it. Both your mind and your body will be glad you did.

9

NATURE'S "BEST SMELLER" AND HOW IT WILL BRING YOU GLOWING GOOD HEALTH

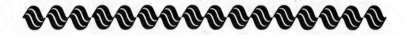

A friend of ours named L. John Harris has a "thing" about garlic. We like garlic too, but not in the way he does. Harris has written *The Book of Garlic*. When you walk into his house you see signs of his obsession everywhere — especially in his kitchen. But, says Harris, the garlic's not just for eating. It's a remedy for almost anything that ails you.

Not only has Harris written a book, he has his own unusual organization Lovers of the Stinking Rose, based in Berkeley, California. The Lovers publish the journal *Garlic Times*. There's very little about garlic you couldn't learn by reading each issue. You might learn more about garlic than you ever want to know, but since Harris agreed to reveal a lot of the secrets of the *Allium sativum* for us, we won't say that. Actually, garlic is a fascinating subject and it's an incredibly potent plant as well.

We have previously told the reader some specific applications for garlic, especially in the chapter on colds.

But if you want to be able to use this simple and versatile plant in the myriad of wonderful ways it can be used, then it is important to look at it in the broadest sense. This simple leek is a virtual cornucopia of health, definitely one of the greatest of the cornerstones of home healing. This is why we are devoting a whole chapter to it. One of the wonderful things about garlic is that to enjoy its medicinal and health benefits, one needn't do much more than take the stuff.

NO-SMELL PILLS

There are garlic pills and capsules available at your local health food store that have the great benefit of being deodorized. It is possible to remove the characteristic garlic smell and yet retain the medicinal values, because what gives the garlic its potent smell luckily doesn't have much to do with its beneficial functions.

THE JAPANESE GARLIC MACHINE

Both Harris' book and *Garlic Times* tell the story of a Japanese firm which markets a large, complicated device, a garlic therapy administering shower, that mixes the bulb with the water descending on the body. The founder of this firm has written a book that has been a "best-smeller" in Japan. He also has thousands of people coming to his Oyama Garlic Laboratory in Amagasaki, Japan every year for treatments that include not only the showers but oral administrations of the wondrous plant.

Despite the pills and showers and so on, the simple, wonderful fact is that you needn't go to Japan or even to the health food store to take advantage of garlic's potent curing powers. All you have to do is cut it up and eat it. However, as you will discover in the next section, you might be well-advised to use a garlic press, a simple, widely available little tool for your kitchen. Then have plenty of garlic on hand.

It isn't appropriate in this book to tell you all the lore of garlic. Suffice to say it is a very rich one — garlic has been recognized as one of man's most potent foods and drugs for centuries. We recommend Harris' book for those who want to delve deeply into its lore, but we will cover a great many of the practical ways of using the bulb.

GARLIC FOR THE HEART

John A. suffered from high blood pressure — high enough that he had to take medication. His blood pressure was the result of being overweight, nothing more. Not all people with high blood pressure are so lucky. His doctor said that if he were to reduce, his blood pressure would consequently go down. And indeed his blood pressure had gone down when his weight had. But in the meanwhile he had to keep using medication; this was something of a shock for a 45-year-old man who had enjoyed good health most of his life.

He had originally gone to the doctor's because he wasn't feeling well. When he found out what the problem was, he felt even worse. But the medication did seem to help; and it quite possibly saved his life. One day, however, he ran out of medication, and didn't take any for three or four days. He didn't know for sure his blood pressure was too high — you can't always tell that it is. But he knew he was beginning to feel the way he had before he began

151

taking the medication. It was not a good weekend to run out of the medication — his doctor was out of town for the next several days.

Thinking of a discussion about garlic John had had not so long before with a friend of his, he took out some cloves of garlic, and did something most people probably would have been wise enough not to do. He chomped down into a clove of garlic. If anyone doesn't believe garlic is potent stuff, they need only to try doing that! Soon John's wife came home and laughed when he told her what he had done. She reached into a drawer and pulled out a hand garlic presser and showed him how to use it. Now this is not scientific proof — we would never recommend using garlic juice instead of the appropriate medication for high blood pressure — but John felt substantially better. He felt as if his blood pressure were coming down. Nowadays John does his best not to miss his regular medication, but as an extra preventive, he also regularly takes garlic. And now he is trying to lose some weight.

EVIDENCE FOR GARLIC

There is scientific evidence that garlic is good for the heart. In Harris' survey, he reports among other things that while in the United States one in three deaths are due to heart disease, in Spain and Italy, where lots of garlic is consumed, the heart disease death rate is much lower. According to figures from the United Nations Demographic Yearbook, only one in seventeen deaths are due to heart disease in Spain. The Italian rate is somewhat worse, but still better than ours. Some other countries with low rates of heart deaths are also big consumers of garlic, such as Korea, the south of France, and certain areas of Russia and other Slavic countries.

In Harris' book, he notes that in an issue of Lancet, the prestigious British medical journal, two top-flight cardiologists did an experiment with ten people, all healthy. One group of five was given extra amounts of garlic juice straight; the other five used an oil extract of the juice. In both cases the results were the same: The cholesterol level, believed to be a major factor in hardening of the arteries, went down considerably.

As was mentioned before, John A. took garlic for what he feared and what felt like, was high blood pressure. Harris reports on a number of different experiments, done all over the world, that demonstrate the ability of garlic to reduce high blood pressure. It would obviously be risky to replace your prescribed medication with garlic for blood pressure, but it also is obvious that extra garlic — or any garlic at all if you haven't been taking any — cannot be bad for your heart.

A GREAT AID TO FASTER HEALING

From his research, Harris found that the raw juice of garlic diluted in water and applied with sphagnum moss as a bandage had been used as an antiseptic in England during World War I. During World War II, the British government purchased thousands of tons of garlic for treating soldiers' wounds, and none of the men so treated had septic poisoning.

WHY IS GARLIC SO POTENT?

When Harris became fascinated with garlic's medicinal values, he wanted to find just what "magic ingredient" gave the bulb so many miraculous healing properties.

It seems, says Harris, that the key to the garlic's amazing ability to fight microbe infections is in its sulphur content. On the other hand, some researchers believe it may just be garlic's vitamin and mineral content that might be the basis of its reputation as a healer. Some of the earliest scientific evidence for the effectiveness of garlic for a variety of ailments came in 1939 from two New York doctors, Edward Kotin and David Stein, who first studied patient complaints and the effectiveness of garlic. They concluded in *The New York Physician:* "An excellent medicament for employment in a diversity of conditions. We believe that the vitamin and mineral factors do much to cause this to be a drug of noteworthy usage."

Garlic's use as both a health aid and a health booster has been known for considerably longer than the present day. Doctors in Elizabethan times prescribed it as an antidote to scurvy, along with the more famous scurvy remedy of limes. Obviously, the effect was produced because of garlic's vitamin C content — though the doctors didn't know that. But to eat garlic for its Vitamin C content in the amounts that Linus Pauling recommends, for example, behooves even so ardent a garlic admirer as Harris to suggest a modern vitamin pill for this.

Harris says while the high vitamin and mineral count in garlic cannot be underestimated, the reason it appears to be so potent a specific for microbes is, again, its high sulphur content. In the Soviet Union a widely used antibiotic is extracted from garlic, and used as a regular medicine. While it is not as powerful as more conventional antibiotics, it seems to be far more effective against certain germs our conventional antibiotics have little effect against, and there is a growing number of these to contend with today. Some of the medical evidence on garlic is truly amazing. In 1950 a German doctor revealed that garlic oil seems to kill organisms that are specifically bad for human beings, and not hurt those that are good for us. Harris points out that a surprising number of researchers have agreed on garlic's value for various stomach disorders, and here again, the reason is that garlic stimulates the production of normal intestinal flora "in opposition to pathogenic bacteria."

SOME MORE GARLIC HEALTH TIPS

Harris has collected numerous tips for health in his pursuit of the greater glory of garlic. Here are some:

Athlete's Foot: When you use whatever commercial ointment you use each day, add some juice of garlic as well.

Dandruff: Some cloves infused in wine or water will eliminate dandruff and perhaps stimulate hair to grow on the top of the head if used as a scalp wash.

Sinus Problems: If you put some garlic cloves into water for an hour and use the water as nose drops, you might be surprised to find that your sinus problem, or runny or stuffy nose, will be a thing of the past.

GARLIC FOR ASTHMA

If you have asthma, you might consider the following case, as given to Harris by a gentleman writing from San Diego, California. This man had been treated with a cortisone drug for a respiratory ailment. He had become, sad to tell, a cortisone addict. Furthermore, he was suffering from glaucoma and sinusitis as side effects of the cortisone. His infections had eventually developed into chronic asthma, and for years he had suffered from misery and hospitalization until he was forced to retire. Then he heard of the garlic cure for asthma. As he slowly tapered off his cortisone medicine, he ate more and more raw garlic bulbs two or three times a day. After several months he was taking only the garlic, and, more importantly, he was not bothered any more by the asthma. Furthermore his glaucoma had receded. The man knew it was the garlic that had accomplished this because whenever he cut back on the garlic, his asthma would begin to reappear. Garlic had given him a new lease on life.

Actually garlic has been recommended for asthma many times before. One herbal expert suggests making a syrup of garlic when using it as a remedy for asthma.

GARLIC WORKS IN THE
WORST OF CIRCUMSTANCES

Did garlic save this man's life? Fred A. from San Luis Obispo, California, wrote Harris his experience with garlic. He believes the reason he survived in a Japanese prisoner of war camp in China during World War II was that every day his Japanese captors gave him a full clove of chopped-up garlic in a glass of water. This went on for two-and-a-half years. He says that as a result of the rough conditions he encountered during those years he lost more than 40 pounds, but he believes that "were it not for this 'rose,' I don't know what my health might be today."

MORE UNIQUE GARLIC REMEDIES

The Best Part for Blood Pressure: One Ozark herbalist who grows and knows a lot about herbs — herbs have been the traditional medicine of the hills for centuries — says she uses the entire garlic bulb as her high blood pressure medicine.

Garden Pests: Another fascinating thing about garlic that amazed us is its ability to protect gardens from harmful pests. Again, this seems to be a case where it seeks out what is bad to man and destroys it, while aiding what is good. Some recipes call for blending garlic and water, straining the liquid through a cheesecloth, and spraying it on plants to get rid of unwanted "guests." Other gardeners have good results from planting a few garlic plants among their other plants. Recent scientific evidence has shown that this tradition has a solid basis, that garlic has insecticide and insect-repellant qualities. It is effective against all pests from malaria mosquitos to houseflies, without having any adverse effects on people, pets or other plants.

Rheumatism: There have been various reports of rheumatism sufferers obtaining relief either by drinking a garlic syrup, or by rubbing the painful joint with cut garlic.

Longevity: There is a long tradition that links longevity with garlic consumption. While such a connection has not yet been scientifically established, the fact that many Bulgarians seem to live well past 100 is interesting, for their habit is to chew garlic often. During the Middle Ages, people who chewed garlic seemed to be the ones who didn't come down with the plague.

So the moral of the story seems to be that garlic, however humble and smelly a thing some people may think it is, is really a plant we should all praise. It is a marvelous little plant that not only can spice up our food so it tastes a million times better, but can remedy specific problems, and improve our overall health many times over. With this new knowledge, you probably won't blanch as much as you might have at one recipe we saw in the *Garlic Times* for garlic-flavored ice cream. Even now, we don't think we're that converted.

ZINC FOR BECOMING A "BEST SMELLER"

Incidentally, if you've been using a lot of garlic recently, and your friends have been making snide comments about it, try taking a couple of zinc tablets. These are guaranteed to make you a "best smeller" again in no time.

SUMMARY

Even though garlic has a bad reputation with some people, if you happen to be one of these people, you ought to consider changing your view of the lowly bulb. For it is a good thing to eat a lot of; it will prevent illnesses and keep you healthier. If you have rebelled all your life against using garlic in your food, now is the time to consider changing that. Garlic really does improve the taste of food — and it is so good for you as well.

But if you find you can't overcome your objections to the smell, take a trip to your health food store to purchase some of the garlic powders, pills, or capsules that have had the smell removed. That way you will get the best of both worlds.

10

A SUBTLE, FAR-REACHING, AND READILY AVAILABLE ORIENTAL VEGETABLE REMEDY

The most amazing single substance that no home should be without is ginseng, "the man root," as the Chinese named it, because its root indeed resembles a human figure. Anyone familiar with Oriental cultures knows about ginseng, for the oddly shaped root is a staple in China, Korea, Japan and Russia, among other places. Taken as a daily tonic, ginseng can enable you to experience life at its optimum, or at least so believe many Asians of all classes and nationalities. It is considered such a cure-all and general elixir that is regarded as absolutely vital by millions of Orientals. Confucius himself praised its medicinal value very highly. One Chinese herbalist never failed to take ginseng in one form or another for all the years of his life, and according to official Chinese government records, this herbalist was 256 years old when he died in 1933. It is thought to rebuild the tissues, dissipate excess and embarrassing gas, ease pain, and give more energy. Thus it is thought to be good for both the healthy and the ill.

AN AUTHENTIC APHRODISIAC

Ginseng has a tradition of being a potent aphrodisiac. In the Soviet Union, ginseng, when administered to a group of men suffering from sterility, dramatically increased their sperm count. More importantly, a small percentage of these men began producing offspring, whereas before they hadn't been able to.

MANY AMAZING CLAIMS

The literature on ginseng is full of amazing claims for cures, sometimes it seems for just about everything that has ever ailed the poor, long-suffering human race. But the ailments it is best known for include coughs, diabetes, indigestion, diarrhea, constipation, lung troubles, urinary tract inflammations, gout, and rheumatism. And if those weren't enough, many Asians use ginseng as an aid for getting to sleep, primarily because the drug has not only tonic values, but sedative effects as well.

GINSENG FOR BEAUTY

Ginseng has been recommended for specific beauty problems — it helps reduce puffiness in the face, for example, if you've been down with the ravages of a cold. In fact, ginseng has become something of a panacea ingredient in most homemade cosmetic remedies — possibly just because it rejuvenates and tones people up. One herbalist we know about through mutual friends is said to use it as a skin conditioner in an herb mixture she puts into her bath. The herbalist also includes comfrey and patchouli in her mix. She believes ginseng is of special value in baths for dry skin. She also uses ginseng in face creams, masks, cleansers and the like, believing that it may be the active ingredient of these things.

FOREIGN RESEARCH SHOWS THE WAY

Despite the fact that only in the last couple of decades has America's medical establishment begun to take ginseng seriously, this plant had a long and successful career in the West in an underground way. Until recently, our medical establishment had simply ignored reports of scientists in other countries that left little doubt that ginseng is indeed a miraculous remedy. New research from several European countries seems to demonstrate that ginseng is a very effective anti-stress remedy, perhaps in part because of its general strengthening effect. In the Soviet Union, ginseng is regarded as an adaptogen. Soviet scientists have isolated 46 folk remedies which "increase non-specific resistance." Of the 46 plants, ginseng was the star of all of them. Few herbs were regarded as true scientific adaptogens, which meant having a "universal defense action." An adaptogen would be both beneficial for specific ailments and also a preventive for healthy people; a true adaptogen like ginseng has a regulating effect. Soviet scientists found that it aided both individuals suffering from mild high as well as low blood pressures. Adaptogens must also have no bad side effects, and yet should provide both a strengthening effect and an all-around resistance-building effect as well. It is recognized that man, by his basic nature, was never meant to deal with the kind of stress that modern life, with its crowded cities, and polluted air and water and food, impose on him. Something like ginseng may offer real hope, because its effects are so wide and well-documented.

GINSENG'S UNUSUAL STIMULANT EFFECT

Also in Russia, ginseng is highly prized, and that country's medical establishment has conducted voluminous tests and spent millions of rubles in researching the subject. Russian scientific research on its own Siberian ginseng reveals that the stuff works very much like a stimulant in that it seems to increase your capacity for work by, among other things, cutting down on fatigue. In one study of a group of Russian workers in a high-stress occupation, ginseng appeared to not only increase the capacity for work dramatically, but it also cut down on mistakes the workers made. Yet unlike most stimulants, ginseng appears to have no bad side effects.

IT'S GOOD FOR THE HEART, AND
PROTECTS YOU IN OTHER WAYS, TOO

In other Soviet experiments on rats, ginseng seemed to offer protection against the ravages of alcohol, which is epidemic in that country, and the toxic side-effects of medical drugs. Another Soviet experiment showed dramatic results when a group of heart patients suffering from arteriosclerosis took ginseng. Still another research case from that same nation demonstrated a very beneficial result on blood sugar level in a diabetes patient.

Generally, Russian research has shown that ginseng stimulates both the physical and mental activities of the body and that it also strengthens and protects the body when it is undergoing severe and/or prolonged physical strain.

166

When Russian astronauts blast off in a space capsule, one of the things they take with them to give them the energy and ability to deal with the rigors of outer space is ginseng.In Siberia, a form of ginseng grows that the Russians believe is just as good as the Chinese variety. The Russians have tried to cultivate ginseng — but it is a plant that is not easy to cultivate.

EARLY AMERICAN EXPERIENCES
WITH GINSENG

Some Indian tribes in colonial America used ginseng; their medicines all came from the earth, and they had had centuries of experience from which to draw. The Iroquois nation used ginseng for as long as has been known; its medicine men believed it carried in it the spirit of previous generations of medicine men. Interestingly, the Iroquois prescribed ginseng root for warriors suffering from "old years' fire."

China claims to grow the best varieties of ginseng, and Korea and the Soviet Union come next. (Ginseng is so important in those countries that the governments of all three nations heavily regulate and guarantee the quality of what is sold. The processing is a complex process, taking as long as 40 days). But ginseng also grew naturally in the United States, especially under the once wide-spread chestnut trees in the hardwood forests that used to dot the East Coast. It took a lot of hunting to find ginseng even back then, however, for ginseng does not grow together under trees in large patches. It is a rather solitary plant. Eventually most of the ginseng that was easy to obtain was harvested. While some purists claim it is not quite as good as Chinese ginseng, Asians have been willing to pay good money for the American stuff for centuries — thus was ginseng the basis of much early East-West trade. In the 1840s, some 640,000 pounds of dried American ginseng was being sent to China each year.

By the late nineteenth century, most of the good wild ginseng was gone. There was a brief flurry of ginseng activity on the west coast, however; Chinese laborers who had come to build the nation's transcontinental railroads discovered ginseng throughout northern California, Oregon and Washington. But in a few short years, these supplies had disappeared from the American continent also.

AN ADAMANT COLONIAL SUPPORTER TELLS HOW GINSENG GAVE HIM MORE ENERGY

One of the early proponents of ginseng in the colonies was William Byrd, who founded a plantation in Virginia, and was also a writer as well. Byrd had a profound distrust of doctors and lived a healthy life of 70 years without them, dying in 1744. He suggested that the best exercise was to walk and chew ginseng root because it not only gave him lots of extra energy, but also far better spirits. Byrd noted that "Its vertues are, that it gives an uncommon Warmth and Vigour to the Blood, and frisks the Spirit beyond any other cordial. It chears the Heart even of a Man that has a bad Wife, and makes him look down with great Composure on the crosses of the World." He claimed that it aided the lungs and the stomach, and strengthened the bowels, and not only makes one live longer, but have a better old age by rendering it "chearful, and good-humor'd."

CHEWING GINSENG

Throughout the colonies, Byrd was not the only one using ginseng. Before the American Revolution, many of the colonists chewed something — and it wasn't necessarily tobacco they were chewing. The colonists used to chew wads of ginseng whenever their stomachs felt bad.

HOW TO OBTAIN GINSENG

Although ginseng is not cheap, it is not really expensive or unavailable. Many forms of it are carried in most health food stores. If you purchase ginseng that displays government stamps from North or South Korea, China, or the Soviet Union on its packaging, you are guaranteed that you are buying the genuine article. Although there are many prices and varieties, some types are believed to have greater curative powers than others for different things, thus making the complete study of ginseng an endlessly fascinating subject. You also won't want to ignore American ginseng. For as we mentioned, it has a long and traditional history, going back to the Indians, and then becoming very much a part of American folk medicine as well. In the Ozarks, people mix ginseng and other herbs with their home brewed whiskey.

HOW TO USE GINSENG

Whatever the kind of ginseng, one thing to keep away from all forms of it is metal. Metal has the power to turn ginseng black and poisonous. If you're going to cut the stuff into bite size pieces, it certainly doesn't hurt to steam the root for five minutes, or until it softens a bit. Generally traditional Chinese medicine believes that if you want to take ginseng for stomach problems, the liquid or powdered form is the best. Pills help best for congestion and chills, according to the traditional ways. If you are really ill, take your ginseng in liquid form, which could even be in a soup. If you're taking ginseng for weak limbs, do so in the morning on an empty stomach. And again, use no metal containers or metal knives in preparing your ginseng, however you take it. Real devotees of ginseng use a lot of it in their cooking. Most Chinese cookbooks should help you here. It is not accidental that the root used in cooking is also the most cited herbal remedy in Chinese medical texts.

Actually, most recent scientific advice we've found suggests that the best way to take your ginseng may also be one of the easiest — in a powdered root form.

ANN R.'S "PICK-ME-UP"

One day Ann R., a teenager, went to visit a friend. Jane was defiantly proud of the fact that she liked hamburgers and white bread and other over-processed foods. But she had to admit to her far more health-conscious friend that she was feeling listless and tired, not well at all. Her friend offered her two cups of ginseng tea. Ann was dubious, but she was ready to try anything. Within minutes after downing a cup of the tea, she felt a rush of energy and well-being. She eventually improved her diet, but she still enjoys the benefits of ginseng tea whenever she feels listless and sluggish.

A SUCCESSFUL BUSINESSMAN'S SECRET

We know a successful publisher in his 60s who has an incredible amount of drive, equal to that of a 30-year-old in his prime of life. If you should get to know this man, who gets up in the morning and jogs around the hills in the East Bay of San Francisco at least five miles, and then eats sparingly but healthily throughout the day, you'd think that that was what did it. But his female companion, a younger, dazzling, person, says that that is only part of his secret. The real truth about our friend, she has confided on more than one occasion, is that on rising and before going to sleep, he chews a bit of ginseng root, the very best that he can find in the Chinatown section of San Francisco. This is the secret behind his tireless energy and youthful appearance.

GINSENG CURES A STUBBORN CASE OF RHEUMATISM

A doctor reported the case of Rick W., a man in his home town in the Midwest who had suffered many years from rheumatism, yet he was only middle-aged. He had gone the rounds of every local doctor, until he finally settled on one practitioner. Now Rick was treated for several weeks by this doctor without any particularly good results. Then the doctor, who had been experimenting recently with ginseng, decided to try some on him. Not only was Rick suffering from rheumatism, but also from distress in his back and bowels. The good doctor did not tell the middle-aged sufferer what his

171

newest medicine was, but he sent him home to try it. Soon Rick returned, saying that he wanted the bottle refilled; whatever it was he was being given, he enthused, had made the rheumatism disappear, as well as the terrible pains in various parts of his innards. The same practitioner also used a combination of ginseng and pineapple for people with bad problems of digestion. In another case — a man who had suffered from a chronic cough — ginseng tea during and in-between meals did the trick, this doctor reported.

SUMMARY

Ginseng is nature's true wonder drug. Widely used throughout the world, it is quickly gaining adherents in the United States. A great tonic and elixir, it is also believed to increase longevity. You would be well advised to begin taking ginseng, in one or more of its various forms, every day.

11

THE ANCIENT ART
OF HERBALISM

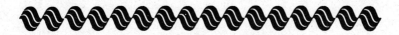

Many of the suggestions in this book, for how to take care of yourself in uncommon ways with things that you never thought could be used as we've suggested, come from the ancient art of herbalism. The use of herbs to cure the common complaints that plague the human race goes back as far as human history. The Greeks and Romans used many herbs, as did most of the peoples of the Orient and our own Native Americans. But it was in Europe in the 16th and 17th centuries that real attempts were made to codify what was known about common healing plants, and how we could use them for our good health. Modern botany and medicine were being born in these centuries. A number of different herbal encyclopedias were written, which have been in the process of being rewritten right up into the twentieth century. As people have been looking more and more for the natural way of doing things, more and more has been written on the subjects of herbs for health.

Generally most doctors are not likely to prescribe

herbs, even though modern drugs — if not compounded directly from plants — are generally comprised of synthetic ingredients based upon plants. But doctors' attitudes are also changing. Many doctors today are themselves switching to more natural medications, and those who haven't gone all the way are using herbals more and more. Today a number of herbs are sold directly in health food stores or at drug stores where "simples" are often kept (simples being the plant parts herbalists believe to be medicinally active), or at your corner drug store in the herb and spice department. Also it would seem wise, when you approach your kitchen in search of better health, to remember Psalm 104:14, "He causeth the grass to grow for the cattle and the herb for the service of man."

USE HERBS WISELY

It is very important that you use herbs carefully. You should choose only the best ones. Currently, there is little federal regulation of the herb industry, although there has been an effort by some of the more responsible herb growers to begin a voluntary policing of the industry. Thus they have formed an Herb Trade Association. Your best protection is probably to find a health food store where you can discuss the different brands there. Some herbs are merely spices that may have medicinal effects, but other are potent medicines. Norman R. Farnsworth, chairman of the department of pharmacology at the University of Illinois Medical Center in Chicago, is one of the nation's top experts on herbs. He has called not only for more intelligent regulation of the herb business, but also government research to establish scientifically just what different herbs do and what their active ingredients are.

In this country we have been behind other countries in herb research; part of the reason is that our mechanized, highly-processed ways of doing things have derided the importance of natural phenomenon such as plants, which is what herbs are. Thus, if you want to research herbs, you must go to the scientific literature on herbs, most of which is from other countries. Not only Dr, Farnsworth, but other reputable herb dealers have asked the government to begin a program of research on the effects of different herbs. Dr. Farnsworth says that at this point the Food and Drug Administration knows so little about herbs they often misspell their names. Until then, the average user must proceed cautiously. In this book, we have tried to stay away from dangerous herbs, although some will obviously be controversial. Sarsaparilla used to be the basis of many old-fashioned root beer concoctions, and it's one of the famous old plants out of American folklore medicine. Yet the government thinks it may have some dangerous side effects. We continue to buy a sarsaparilla drink at our local health food store nonetheless. Herbs are a wonderful thing to study and to buy for your kitchen. They are a fascinating hobby — but one that must be approached carefully and intelligently. On the other hand, they will reward you with more health and a better life. Your kitchen will then become not only a place from which nutrition comes, but also a place from which health flows directly.

HOW DANDELIONS CURED A DOCTOR
OF LIVER TROUBLE

Doctor C., of San Francisco, was afflicted with liver complaints, and in trying to find relief, he had visited doctors in other parts of the country, after trying everything he knew on himself first. Unfortunately the doctors seemed no more able to help him, even though they were supposed to be great specialists. Now Dr. C. was normally not given to using herbs in his own practice; he was very dubious about them. But since nothing anyone had done had helped him, his ears perked up one day when he heard about dandelions, the old herbal remedy for liver complaints. He merely boiled the dried flowers in water, then drank a cupful of the strained liquid several times a day. Doctor C. said he could trace the day his liver complaints ended from the day he first started using dandelions. The pain began to subside after his first dose of the dandelion liquid. Naturally, he began using dandelions as a remedy for his patients suffering from liver trouble — and after nearly two decades of practice, he insisted that almost every one of his patients with a liver complaint got quick relief.

There's nothing exotic about the plant that Dr. C. used so successfully for himself and his patients. Any gardener knows how healthy and hardy dandelions are. We have heard of people who eat dandelions like spinach — they boil and serve the leaves with butter or use the fresh leaves in their salads. The French eat dandelions in sandwiches as a matter of course. Dandelions are also not an uncommon component of coffee substitutes. You can usually buy these in health food stores, but you can also make one yourself. Roast the dandelion roots slowly in your oven, then pulverize with a mortar and pestle or in a blender or food processor. Mix the powder in hot water, whatever amount your taste buds will allow.

AMAZING PARSLEY TEA

Another kind of tea that has helped people with a variety of ailments is made from the lowly parsley, that innocuous little plant that garnishes so many meals. Take a quart of boiling water and a cup of packed fresh parsley and steep for 15 minutes. Strain and put in the refrigerator. Parsley tea seems to have especially helped men suffering from prostate problems, and in general any kidney, liver or bladder problems. There have also been reports that it helps certain varieties of rheumatic pain as well. Take half a cup three times a day for as long as needed. Parsley tea has been used by women suffering from menstrual cramps; digestive pains also often yield to it. Probably because parsley is high in Vitamin A, it has been recommended for eye problems as well.

CHLOROPHYLL AS A DEODORANT

Chlorophyll is one of the most abundant substances on earth. It is the green substance produced by plants when the sun hits them, and it is not only the key to the way plants store the sun's energy, it is what makes them green. Chlorophyll can make you smell sweet, without a lot of unpleasant chemicals, and it is available in almost all health food stores. The reason it is known that chlorophyll can make you smell good, was a long series of experiments that were conducted in 1950 by Dr. F. Howard Westcott. In his first series of tests, he found that chlorophyll reduced detectable underarm odors in a group of five young ladies by nearly 100 percent. Dr. Westcott conducted another, later series of tests on another group of 12 coeds, having them run, and then checking their mouth odors. Since then, Dr. Westcott has continued his experiments, and the result is always the same. Body odors decreased by some 90 percent when his subjects each morning consumed a tablet containing 100 milli-grams of a chlorophyll extract.

TAKE CHIA AND SEE

Most good health food stores carry chia seeds, which are made from nothing more exotic than a variety of sage. Ground chia seeds are an excellent addition to soup and salads or to omelettes; try a sprinkling mixed into your omelette just before you take it out of the pan Chia seeds were widely used by the Indians, and one of the Montezumas took chia seeds in lieu of taxes. Too bad Uncle Sam isn't so wise. An early study of California Indians noted that, on forced 24 hour marches, what kept the noble hunters going was nothing more than a pinch of chia seeds. So when you need endurance, the chia seed is something you should consider.

AN ONION A DAY MIGHT
KEEP THE DOCTOR AWAY

Our good friend L. John Harris has been threatening for a long time to follow up his garlic book with an opus on onions. *The Garlic Times* has even begun seeking onion lore, onion lovers, and assorted other onion facts. But while both onions and garlic are members of the same plant family, it must be admitted that the garlic has the edge. Nonetheless, we have turned up a number of good uses for the noble onion, and we herewith include them.

• If you jam a digit in a door (it can be on either the foot or the hand), try this as a remedy. This will be much more appealing if you can get someone else to do it, since you'll probably be in terrible pain. Pulp some onion, add lots of extra salt, and make a poultice to apply to the wounded digit. Have a friend or a spouse or your child do this while you're sitting there in pain. You'll discover that the pain literally disappears after you apply the poultice.

• Almost any kind of external wound, from bruising to burns, from sores to boils, up to and even including warts, will improve with the addition of chopped raw onions on a poultice such as the one described above. Brown spots and other such blemishes can often be removed from the skin by mixing a teaspoon of onion juice with two teaspoons of vinegar and using the resulting mixture as a wash. A slice of onion placed on top of an insect sting will also afford great relief.

• Onion tea acts as a mild diuretic. Diuretics are what people take when, for one reason or another, they want to rid their body of excess water. (People who want to temporarily lose a little weight or those who suffer from high blood pressure might consider onion tea.) You make onion tea by boiling an onion, needless to say. The leftover water is the tea. Some European doctors have even taken advantage of the onion's diuretic effect and used a regimen of onion tea when the diuretic effect was clearly needed for their patients suffing from bad heart problems.

• To get rid of athlete's foot, try rubbing onion juice between the toes four or five times a day until the horrible disease recedes. A remedy for removing calluses from the feet calls for cutting fresh onions in half, steeping them in strong wine vinegar for four hours, and applying them to the calluses, bound with a kerchief and left overnight. In the morning the calluses can be scraped away, after which it is recommended you give your feet a bath, not for any medicinal reason, but for social reasons.

• To go to sleep with. A well-known family physician some years ago had a unique method for going to sleep.

Here is what he said: "If I am much pressed with work and feel that I am not disposed to sleep, I eat two or three small onions and the effect is magical."

• For reason having nothing to do with medical ones, your family physician may not be inclined to agree with this recommendation. But the fact is that if you suffer from asthma or any kind of bronchial problem, your problems will be considerably helped if you make sure you eat plenty of sliced, raw onions.

• Last but not least, neither of us suffers from bad hearing, and we haven't heard any confirmation of this from our good friend Harris, but we hear that a mixture of two ounces of garlic and onion juice in the ear each day will help cure even some forms of deafness.

HOW COMFREY CURED A
CASE OF ASTHMA

One day a fellow in who had been a long-time sufferer from asthma was visiting another friend who had a comfrey plant in his front yard. Rather absent-mindedly, this sufferer began to nibble on a leaf from the plant. That evening when he got home, he had one of the most pleasant nights he had had in a long time, for he suffered from no asthma. Amazed at this, he decided to try to figure out what different had happened to him that day. He carefully made up lists, and went over everything he did, which included everything he had eaten. He was about to give up in absolute disgust when he remembered standing in front of his friend's house, chewing on that plant. "Perhaps it was those leaves," he thought. So he went back to his friend's to get some more leaves, and since that day he has suffered from asthma no more.

SUMMARY

This book has told you about many remedies for many different ailments and conditions. They can be used in the privacy of your own home. This book is telling you about remedies that you might even have on your kitchen shelf at this very moment. Herbs are related to foods, of course; one of the difficulties the government has had in regulating herbs is that many of them are nothing more than foods or spices. Yet that doesn't mean they can't be potent remedies as well. Herbal remedies are myriad and fascinating, and if we do no more than introduce you to the subject in this volume, that will be accomplishment enough. Try some of the remedies in this book; most are available at any good health food store.

12

MORE UNUSUAL REMEDIES
YOU CAN USE AT HOME

By now you no doubt have a good understanding of the many amazing remedies right at your fingertips, available either around your house or in your local supermarket. Speaking of other readily available health remedies, it is interesting to note how many health writers look upon diet or nourishment as a health remedy in and of itself. Some health experts recommend a strictly vegetarian diet, some a diet of raw foods, others a diet which excludes dairy products and animal fats — but the one concept which runs through almost every health writer's books is that your diet is the first thing to look to when you are trying to improve your health. This is a notion with which both authors of this book heartily concur. While neither of us is a vegetarian or any other kind of food extremist, we do believe that "we are what we eat."

187

AN OPTIMUM PERSONALIZED DIET
FOR GOOD HEALTH

We hope that, as you have read this book, you have realized that the blueprint for good health and a long life that will work best for you is one which you formulate yourself.

With a little information under your belt, so to speak, you can create a diet that will work for you, whether you want to lose weight, maintain your present weight or just feel healthier and more vital. You don't need to buy all your food at an expensive health food store or limit your diet to soy beans and alfalfa sprouts, either.

The key to formulating your own optimum diet is to take inventory of your present diet. Sit down for a quiet hour with paper and pencil. Make a list of everything you presently eat for breakfast, lunch and dinner as well as snacks. It may surprise you a little when you look over the list. Do you see lots of "junk food" lurking there — cookies, pastries, candy, fast food from stands or coffee shops? Modern life tends to make us all much more familiar with the meal-on-the-run than we should be.

Now think a little about your eating patterns and habits. When do you eat your main meal of the day? Most of you will probably answer "At dinnertime." If you're one of those who is hoping to lose weight, you may want to shift the bulk of your eating to earlier in the day, since food consumed after five p.m. tends to lie in the stomach longer without being assimilated as rapidly.

The female half of this writing team made a fascinating discovery not too many years ago while trying to shed a few unwanted pounds. She had been dieting strenuously — nothing but the leanest meat, a few steamed vegetables, no butter, sugar or salt, and no alcohol or desserts. But although she stuck strictly to her diet for several weeks, she hadn't lost enough weight to justify the misery of her diet!

Then on a trip away from home she began eating a large breakfast and cutting down on the amount she ate at dinner accordingly. Within days, she had lost six pounds, just by changing the time of day she ate her main meal! Prior to this discovery, she had been saving up her daily food allotment for dinnertime, and eating most of it then.

Later she discovered that such prestigious weight reduction organizations as Schick Center recommend to their weight loss patients that they eat in an "inverted pyramid" — most of their food intake in the morning at breakfast, a medium-sized lunch at noon and a very small dinner, eaten before four-thirty in the afternoon if possible. The reason for this is that the body tends to metabolize its caloric intake more efficiently when you first get up. You also have a tendency to utilize the most calories when your energy level is high. A hearty breakfast will supply you with the calories you need to "get up and get at 'em" — while a skimpy breakfast of a prefabricated pastry and a cup of coffee grabbed from the catering truck at work will leave you feeling sluggish and unmotivated long before lunchtime rolls around.

By "hearty" we don't mean non-nutritious, of course. If you're trying to lose weight, you will have to cut your calorie intake as well as increase your exercise., But if you've been trying to lose weight on a diet of celery sticks and beef bouillon and haven't seen much success, at least try shifting your main meal to breakfast time before you give up the ship. Eat whatever you feel comfortable eating, but be sure that it is as natural and as close to its original form as possible (i.e., fresh fruits, whole grains, etc.). You may find after a few days that dieting is not only livable, but also very effective!

"FRIENDLY" AND "UNFRIENDLY" FOODS

When you look at the list of foods you often eat and enjoy, do you see many pre-packaged items such as potato chips, soft drinks and pastries? These, we're sorry to say, are the very epitome of "unfriendly" foods. At best, these nutritionless cardboard morsels do nothing to improve your health — at worst, they can make you feel tired, irritable and run-down without your ever suspecting the cause.

There is one area in which we agree with the most extreme health writers: white sugar and refined flour are Public Food Enemies No. 1 and 2 — not necessarily in that order. Refined flour — the "white" flour used to make pastries, pie and most commercial bread you find on supermarket shelves — is a denatured product, used more for the convenience of the manufacturer than for your well-being. Even so-called "whole wheat" bread is often made from white flour with some brown sugar or other coloring added to stimulate a whole-wheat appearance. Real whole-wheat flour, and the bread made from it, is truly the "staff of life"; it is rich in the B vitamins and in some minerals, as well as a host of other nutrients. When you consider that most "fast food" you consume consists primarily of white flour and miscellaneous chemicals, you can begin to realize why you may feel inclined to eat more than you should — there's not much nutrition in refined flour and chemicals, and maybe your body is trying to tell you something.

Likewise, white sugar is every bit the villain it is always painted as being. It does everything from upsetting your blood sugar balance to causing tooth decay, and without further elaboration we should immediately put it high on the list of "unfriendly" foods. If your diet contains anything more than an occasional dose of white sugar — it shouldn't.

So what are the "friendly" foods that will help keep your weight at its optimum level and give you plenty of energy and high spirits? In a nutshell — whole foods, or foods as close to their original state as possible. This means fresh fruits and vegetables, nuts, grains, dairy products without preservatives or other dubious additions, and a relatively low proportion of beef and pork to chicken, turkey and fish. An occasional glass of wine with dinner will probably not do you any harm, but more than one or two drinks a day is not going to help your health much and it will make it harder for you to lose weight. Basically, that's all you have to remember about "friendly" and "unfriendly" foods and, indeed, about the whole diet question. Just use your own common sense when it comes to selecting the components of your meals — try to avoid "fast food" whenever possible — and do try to make your morning meal the biggest meal of the day. You will, if you follow these simple suggestions, find that your kitchen can be one of your most powerful allies in the search for better health and a nicer-looking you.

FOR LADIES ONLY

The next few health tips will be primarily for you female readers. There has been a revolution in cosmetics during the last few years, as you probably suspect if you've been reading the papers. Many women are becoming increasingly alarmed at the number of potentially hazardous substances found in commercial makeup and skin care preparations available in drug and department stores. Also, more and more women are beginning to appreciate the wonder-working powers of natural cosmetics.

In the last few years it has become possible to purchase so-called "organic" cosmetics in health food stores and in some more conventional shops as well, but when you find how easy it is to make some of these concoctions at home for only a few pennies, you probably won't want to spend the money. Then, too, you will know exactly what your homemade natural cosmetics contain if you make them yourself. Remember that these natural cosmetics can be assembled using ingredients you have around the house, or can easily get at the supermarket or, in a few cases, at a drugstore or health food store.

NATURE'S OWN COSMETIC — THE AVOCADO

It was believed for many years that nutrients could not be absorbed through the skin. Then, at the end of World War II, thousands of emaciated victims in Nazi concentration camps were rescued from the gas chambers only to be doomed, apparently, by severe malnutrition. But the "impossible" happened — many of those prisoners, so near starvation that their systems simply could not assimilate food, were saved when nutrients were massaged into their skin.

These days, topically-applied vitamins have become

therapeutic agents for a wide variety of ills ranging from acne to serious burns. It has even been shown that often, when you want to get vitamins to a particular spot on the skin, topical applications are more effective than ingestion by mouth.

This brings us to the avocado, that familiar green fruit (often mistakenly called a vegetable) that not only makes some delicious dishes, but is also one of the most remarkable natural cosmetics.

One of the world's finest skin nutrients, the avocado is a powerhouse of vitamins, minerals, and life-giving properties that can do your body a great deal of good, outside as well as inside.

PROTECTING YOUR SKIN
FROM SUN DAMAGE

As a defense against sun damage to the skin, the oil of the avocado is both a highly effective lubricant and the most efficient natural oil in the plant world when it comes to screening out ultraviolet radiation from the sun or other sources.

This fact was known to the early Indians of the California and Mexican deserts. These Indians would break open the fruit and smear the interior pulp all over their bodies as protection against the harsh rays of the desert sun. You can do the same if you want to keep your skin young and smooth in the process of acquiring a tan.

But the real beauty of the avocado lies in its moisturizing abilities. The flesh and oil of the avocado are humectant — they draw water to themselves, and hold it there, thus keeping your skin as dewy and as youthful as it was when you were a babe in arms.

193

AN AVOCADO RECIPE FOR SUPER SKIN

Here is an easily-made concoction which combines the avocado and wheat germ oil for a super facial cocktail: Puree the flesh of half an avocado in a blender or food processor, then stir in a tablespoon of wheat germ oil (available at any health food store). Rub this mixture into the neck and jawline with firm strokes, and leave on half an hour, or longer, such as overnight, for even better results. You will find that flabby jawlines, sagging facial muscles, wrinkles and crepey necks will respond beautifully to this super "skin bomb"! The mixture will keep for about three days as long as it is refrigerated in an airtight container. If you still have some of it left after three days, discard it and make a fresh batch.

The flesh of the avocado can also be used by itself as suggested above as a skin moisturizer, or it can be combined with various ingredients to make other types of facial masks or treatments.

Avacado/Honey/Yogurt Facial Scrub: Beat the pulp of a large, fresh avocado until it is mushy, then add a few tablespoons of pure, unfiltered honey and half a cup of plain yogurt. Mix together. Pat mixture onto face and neck with cotton balls or pads. Leave on for a few minutes, or as long as half an hour for super-cleansing. Rinse off; towel dry. This is an excllent mixture to use if you have blackheads or other skin blemishes.

Avocado Oily Skin Mixture: Mix the pulp of one avocado with two or three tablespoons of freshly-squeezed lemon juice. Apply as above. You can also mix the avocado with pure cider vinegar for oily skin and other skin blemish problems. Use three tablespoons of vinegar. (This mixture is stronger than the lemon juice mixture, but since it should be left on for longer periods if you require thorough cleansing, those who aren't fond of the smell of vinegar may want to use the lemon juice version and leave it on a little longer — say, forty-five minutes).

Avocado Dry Skin Remedy: For dry skin in areas such as elbows, cut an avocado in half and remove the pulp. Rub the skin against the affected area.

MORE NATURAL COSMETICS
YOU CAN MAKE AT HOME

While we're on the subject of natural food-based beauty aids, let's look at that old standby yogurt. You probably think of yogurt as a healthy snack or a low-calorie substitute for sour cream, but did you know that it is also an incredible skin beautifier as well? The friendly bacteria which originally transform milk into yogurt create an acid balance which makes yogurt ideal for toning and firming your face.

For oily skin, combine equal parts fresh, unprocessed plain yogurt and cider vinegar. Dab on with cotton balls to wipe the oily spots on your face, omitting the under-eye area. Do this every night before going to bed, as well as when you put on your makeup in the morning. You will see tighter pores and a fresh glow in a week or less.

If you dislike the smell of vinegar, equal parts of yogurt and fresh, unfiltered honey will also work wonders to cleanse and tone your face. Use as above. This mixture is a little less drying than the vinegar-yogurt mixture.

A FURTHER SOLUTION TO THE
"OIL WELL" PROBLEM

It is amazing how many of us suffer from oily skin, even when we are long past the age of acne. But most likely, our "oil wells" tend to be located in specific areas of our faces, with the other areas being dry or normal. To cleanse these "oil wells," rub the areas with the juice from a freshly-squeezed lemon. This will mop up the oil that causes blackheads and pimples without affecting the pH balance of the rest of the face.

BARBARA C.'S NATURAL TIP
FOR BEAUTIFUL HAIR

A friend of ours, Barbara C., is a makeup artist in Hollywood who is very enthusiastic about natural cosmetics. She uses them frequently in her makeup studio. One of her favorite tricks to add body and volume to her hair is to add two egg whites and a generous dash of freshly squeezed lemon juice to her shampoo when she washes her hair. She claims that her hair is naturally rather thin and lackluster, but you'd never suspect it from looking at her.

PLANTS THAT CAN MAKE YOU
LOOK RAVISHING

Here are a couple of plant cosmetic concoctions that you might try. The plants can often be found growing near where you live, in vacant lots and on roadsides.

Dandelion Skin Toner: Gather a large handful of dandelion flowers; simmer them in two cups of water for ten or fifteen minutes, then let cool. Strain the liquid through cheesecloth and apply to the skin. After it has dried, rinse off. This dandelion liquid will tone and balance your skin and increase the circulation.

Sorrel Leaf Face and Skin Wash: Sorrel is a perennial plant often found growing in vacant lots and other areas where grass and weeds grow wild. Over the years, the leaves of this plant have been used as a mouthwash and gargle; nowadays it is seen more and more in fine cooking as an ingredient in soups and salads.

To make a face and skin wash with sorrel leaves, gather the leaves when they are fresh. Put about a cupful of carefully washed leaves into a large bowl or other non-metallic vessel and pour three cups of boiling water over them. When mixture has cooled, strain through cheesecloth. Using cotton balls, dab the liquid gently on the face and neck. It will cleanse your skin thoroughly but gently.

A HANDY REFERENCE GUIDE
TO HOME COSMETICS

The following guide will tell you what particular substance to use for oily or dry skin, or for that common condition, "combination skin."

Dry Skin: Natural vegetable oils, such as olive and soybean oil. Use cold-pressed oils only. Avocado pulp. Natural cocoa butter is a good sunscreen.

Oily Skin: Corn oil. Safflower oil. Witch hazel (available at any drugstore). Cider vinegar. Rosewater (also available at drugstores, or in stores that specialize in Middle Eastern or other ethnic foods).

Combination Skin Conditions: Honey. Yogurt. Wheat germ oil. Citrus juices such as lemon and orange.

The various substances can be combined in any form you wish to use, as long as you don't mix oily skin and dry skin substances together. These concoctions can also be added to your bath water, along with aromatic herbs, dried flower petals, or spices, for a super natural bath.

A FEW FINAL NATURAL REMEDIES

Finally, here are a few natural remedies for miscellaneous ailments. As one of our mothers used to remark, "It's always those miscellaneous ailments that are the hardest to beat." To which we can only add, "Amen." But these easy-to-use home treatments might do the job.

Natural Cough Syrup: Chop up a couple of medium-sized onions. Mix with a half-cup of pure, unfiltered honey. Place in the top half of a double boiler and cook down until mixture resembles a thick syrup. Take a teaspoonful of the cough syrup every hour if your cough is severe; it seems to work more efficiently if it is warmed before you take it. Garlic and honey are also good when there is a lot of phlegm trapped in your chest, or if your cough has affected your bronchial tubes, or in cases where you have been coughing and spitting up for long periods of time.

Rheumatism Relief: Chop into dice, but do not peel, a pound of potatoes. Place in five cups of water and bring to boil. Continue boiling until half of the water has evaporated. When the liquid has cooled down, dip a washcloth or some cheesecloth in it and sponge the affected parts.

Hiccup Eliminator: Soak a whole sugar cube in freshly-squeezed lemon juice. Let dissolve in the mouth. If needed, repeat.

Chilblain Alleviator: Mash a roasted or boiled turnip until soft. While it is still hot, apply to the soles of the feet and tie with a bandage. Repeated applications over a few days are recommended in especially severe or painful cases.

AND LAST BUT NOT LEAST,
BEWARE THE FULL MOON

It's true. If one of your regular conditions is acting up — ulcers are an example, or chest pains — look outside and you shouldn't be surprised to discover that a full moon is looming over the horizon. A number of studies have established a relationship between an increase in arson, violent crimes, and strange behavior in mental hospitals when the moon is full. Now Ralph Morris, a professor of pharmacology at the University of Illinois's medical center, has concluded a study showing that health problems also become more severe under the full moon. Morris suggests that people with problems like bleeding ulcers and chest pains make doubly sure they are taking their medications.

SUMMARY

We hope that you have enjoyed reading this book as much as we have enjoyed writing it. We are sure that you will be able to make good use of a number of the unusual remedies included in this chapter, and in all the other chapters as well. Good health to you!

INDEX